Nephron-sparing Surgery

Nephron-sparing Surgery

Edited by

KRISHNA PILLAI SASIDHARAN MS MCh
Professor and Head
Department of Urology
Kasturba Medical College
Karnataka, India

MARK S SOLOWAY MD
Professor and Chairman
Department of Urology
Miller School of Medicine
University of Miami
Miami, FL, USA

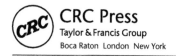

CRC Press
Taylor & Francis Group
Boca Raton London New York

CRC Press is an imprint of the
Taylor & Francis Group, an **informa** business

CRC Press
Taylor & Francis Group
6000 Broken Sound Parkway NW, Suite 300
Boca Raton, FL 33487-2742

© 2008 by Taylor & Francis Group, LLC
CRC Press is an imprint of Taylor & Francis Group, an Informa business

First issued in paperabck 2019

No claim to original U.S. Government works

ISBN 13: 978-0-367-44618-5 (pbk)
ISBN 13: 978-1-84184-636-1 (hbk)

Visit the Taylor & Francis Web site at
http://www.taylorandfrancis.com

and the CRC Press Web site at
http://www.crcpress.com

Contents

Contributors

Rajinikanth Ayyathurai MD MRCS(Ed)
Department of Urology
Miller School of Medicine
University of Miami
Miami, FL
USA

Larry W Belbeck
Professor
Department of Pathology and Molecular Medicine
McMaster University
Hamilton, Ontario
Canada

Saleh Binsaleh MD FRCS(C)
Clinical Fellow
Laparoscopy and Endourology
McMaster University
Department of Surgery (Urology)
Hamilton, Ontario
Canada

Vincent G Bird MD
Assistant Professor of Urology
Miller School of Medicine
University of Miami
Miami, FL
USA

Arun Chawla MD
Clinical Fellow
Urology and Renal Transplant
McMaster University
Hamilton, Ontario
Canada

Ashis Chawla MD FRCS(C)
Clinical Fellow, Laparoscopy and Endourology
Centre for Minimal Access Surgery (CMAS)
Section of Urology, Department of Surgery
McMaster University
Hamilton, Ontario
Canada

Kathy Chorneyko MD
Department of Pathology
St Joseph's Healthcare
Hamilton, Ontario
Canada

Anil Kapoor MD FRCSC
Associate Professor of Surgery (Urology)
Diplomate, American Board of Urology
Program Director, Urologic Laparoscopy
Centre for Minimal Access Surgery (CMAS)
Surgical Director, Renal Transplantation
Director, Urologic Research Group
McMaster Institute of Urology at St Joseph's
  Healthcare
Juravinski Cancer Center
McMaster University
Hamilton, Ontario
Canada

Bruce R Kava MD
Chief, Urology Service
Department of Veterans Affairs Medical Center
Miami, FL
USA

Ming-Kuen Lai MD
Professor, Department of Urology
National Taiwan University Hospital
Taipei
Taiwan

Raymond J Leveillee MD
Associate Professor of Clinical Urology
Department of Urology
Miller School of Urology
University of Miami
Miami, FL
USA

Murugesan Manoharan MD FRCS(Eng) FRACS(Urol)
Associate Professor of Urologic Oncology
Director, Neobladder and Urostomy Centre
University of Miami School of Medicine
Miami, FL
USA

Kumaresan Natarajan MS FRCS(Ire) FRCS(Edin) DNB MCh
Associate Professor
Department of Urology
Kasturba Medical College
Karnataka
India

Alan M Nieder MD
Assistant Professor of Urology
Miller School of Medicine
University of Miami
Miami, FL
USA

Krishna Pillai Sasidharan MS MCh
Professor and Head
Department of Urology
Kasturba Medical College
Karnataka
India

Mark S Soloway MD
Professor and Chairman
Department of Urology
Miller School of Medicine
University of Miami
Miami, FL
USA

Marshall S Wingo
Department of Urology
Miller School of Medicine
University of Miami
Miami, FL
USA

Preface

The concept of this book on nephron-sparing surgery germinated almost two years ago in an interaction at the European Association of Urology annual conference held in Istanbul between one of the editors and Mr Alan Burgess, Senior Publisher, of Informa Healthcare. The need for an elaborate book encompassing all the strategic facets of nephron-sparing surgery, a resurgent topic of import, was palpably evident to both.

Evidently, a project of this kind has to be essentially collaborative in character. Hence, the editors sought and readily obtained support from chosen authors from four major global universities, namely University of Miami, USA, McMaster University, Canada, National Taiwan University, and Manipal University, India.

The general layout of chapters of the book is so designed to focus on those areas related to actual performance of nephron-sparing surgery. The chapters 'Hypothermia and renoprotective measures in nephron-sparing surgery' and 'Evaluation of energy sources used in nephron-sparing surgery' belong to that genre. We have also widened the compass of the book by including chapters related to relevant issues such as renal anatomy, pathology of renal cell carcinoma, and renal imaging.

This text is not a mere compilation of already known facts, nor is it an elaborate review of the current literature. It is much more than that. All contributors to this volume without exception are either involved in the practice of nephron-sparing surgery routinely or in work in related spheres. The contributors, therefore, suffuse their respective treatises with a wealth of personal experience and perceptions. In a volume of encyclopedic dimension such as this, we do not overlook the fact that some segments of the principal topic are evaluated and discussed in more than one chapter. Such reiteration may be salutary in the sense that it amplifies the width and depth of readers' perceptions about some of the critical areas of nephron-sparing surgery.

We are indebted to many who rendered such excellent support in the making of this tome. It is difficult to pick out a few from so many, and yet it would be churlish not to express our obligation to Dr Anil Kapoor of McMaster University, Dr M Manoharan of University of Miami, and Dr K Natarajan of Manipal University for orchestrating the book-related efforts at their respective ends. We are also beholden to Messrs Alan Burgess and Oliver Walter of Informa Healthcare for overseeing with all commitment publication-related matters and restricting the gestation period of the publication to reasonable limits.

It is our privilege to dedicate this compendium to those surgical craftsmen of yesteryear as well as of the modern era who incessantly strived to define the nephron-sparing concept and let it evolve to assume its present contours.

Krishna Pillai Sasidharan
Mark S Soloway

1

Nephron-sparing surgery: history and evolution

Krishna Pillai Sasidharan

One of the fascinating developments in recent years in the realm of renal cancer management has been the steady ascendancy of nephron-sparing surgery as a therapeutic arm. It is no longer considered a tentative surgical option, but a validated surgical principle designed to fetch long-term, cancer-free survival in organ-confined disease. Currently, its role in the management of advanced renal and metastatic disease is also being increasingly probed.

Interestingly, nephron-sparing surgery is not a modern concept. Its application for localized kidney disease was apparently evident in the late nineteenth century. It is, perhaps, appropriate to review the history of renal surgery in the preceding years to perceive the evolution of the nephron-sparing concept in the proper light.

Gustav Simon is credited with the first planned nephrectomy, which he successfully performed in 1869 to redeem a urinary fistula (Figure 1.1). In the following year he also undertook the first deliberate partial renal resection for hydronephrosis.[1] Simon's successful surgical feats, no doubt, prompted his surgical contemporaries to resort to nephrectomy on a regular basis. Culled data from the early literature disclose that more than 100 cases of nephrectomy were collected up to 1882, 235 by 1886, and more than 300 before 1900 (55 for tumors) in Europe and the United States combined. This period also witnessed the speedy dissemination and practice of the revolutionary concept of Lister's antiseptic surgery. The diffuse application of Lister's principles resulted in a palpable decline in the prevailing surgical morbidity and mortality and expanded the frontiers of renal surgery. These developments helped to anchor nephrectomy more firmly on the pedestal of acceptance and there were no discernible attempts to essay nephron-sparing exercises during that period.

Historically, the first ever nephron-sparing effort was rather inadvertent, when in 1984 Wells extirpated a third of a kidney during enucleation of a perirenal fibrolipoma. Three years later Czerny performed the first documented planned partial resection of a renal tumor (for angiosarcoma), precisely 18 years after the first nephrectomy by Simon[1] (Figure 1.2). In the last quarter of the nineteenth century, it appears there were fervent efforts to define the role of partial resection for localized kidney disease spearheaded by Tillman, Tuffier, Bardenheur, and others. They undertook extensive experimental studies spaning from 1879 to 1900 to probe renal repair mechanisms, compensatory hypertrophy, and the quantum of renal tissue necessary for life after partial resection.[2] However, frequent intraoperative and postoperative complications such as hemorrhage and refractory urinary fistula subdued their surgical fervor for partial renal excision and its application significantly declined during that period and in subsequent years.

The beginning of the twentieth century saw a revival of renal conservation, but it was mostly earmarked for benign clinical situations like cysts, benign tumefactions, and localized hydronephrosis. In 1903 Gregorie performed the first *en bloc* excision of a tumor-harboring kidney along with its fatty capsule, adrenal gland, and adjacent lymph nodes.[1] Gregorie's deft surgical feat had almost all the components of a modern classical radical nephrectomy and it helped to cement, in no uncertain manner, the procedure's validity as a therapeutic option for the management of renal cancer. Total nephrectomy, therefore, prospered for a considerable length of time as the sole effective treatment for malignant kidney tumor.

Rosenstein, however, in 1932 performed partial nephrectomy to palliate a case of kidney cancer and demonstrated its feasibility in cases of renal cancer in which the contralateral kidney's functional capability was suspect: the first unambiguous expression of the relative indication for nephron-sparing surgery.

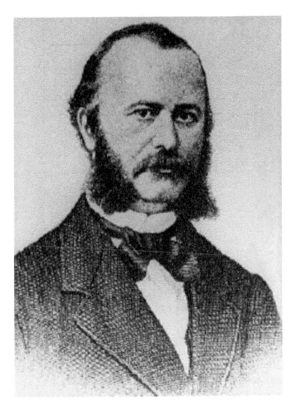

Figure 1.1 Gustav Simon (1824–1876) performed the first planned nephrectomy in 1869 and the first partial nephrectomy in 1870.

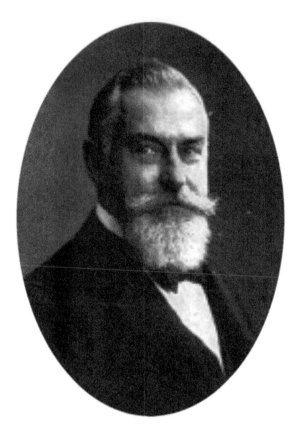

Figure 1.2 Vincenz Czerny (1842–1915) performed the first partial nephrectomy for a renal tumor in 1887.

In 1937 Goldstein and Abeshouse reviewed 296 cases of partial renal resection from the literature (1901–1935), of which 21 were done for malignant tumors.[3] There was only one death and the rest of the nephron-sparing efforts were singularly bereft of major complications such as reactionary hemorrhage or urinary fistula. They prophetically commented that 'small tumors and tumors of moderate size situated at one of the poles of the kidney, may be removed by partial resection out of necessity, but is contra-indicated if the opposite kidney was healthy.' It should be noted that these intrepid and pioneering surgeons continued to perform nephron-sparing surgery, though sporadically, during a period marked by staunch general commitment to nephrectomy as the primary treatment of choice for renal cancer and a belief that partial nephrectomy was more daunting and problem-ridden.

In 1950 Vermooten published a significant paper titled 'Indications for conservative surgery in certain renal tumors: a study based on the growth pattern of the clear cell carcinoma,' and clearly enunciated the ground rules for imperative, relative, and elective indications.[4] Many contemporary pathologic studies notably by Bell[5] highlighting the favorable biologic characteristics of small tumors, particularly their limited metastatic potential, had possibly impacted Vermooten and goaded him into renal conservation. He opined that 'There are certain instances when, for the patient's well being, it is unwise to do a nephrectomy, even in the presence of a malignant growth involving the kidney. The question is whether such a procedure is ever justifiable when the opposite kidney is normal. I am inclined to think that in certain circumstances it may be,' a statement loaded with prophetic overtones. Vermooten was the first to insist that tumors should be excised with a 1 cm margin to discourage local recurrence.

Despite Vermooten's passionate espousal of the concept of nephron-sparing surgery, its advocacy found meager support in the next two decades. During this period (from 1950 to 1967) Zinman and Dowd were able to collate data on only about 18 cases of partial nephrectomy, and appended three of their own. The notable performers of elective nephron-sparing surgery included Badenoch (1950), Ortega (1951), Dufour (1951), Szendroi and Babics (1955), and Hanely (1962). Semb, in 1955, highlighted his operative technique of partial resection.[6]

Robson's landmark articles published in 1963 and 1969 disclosed very convincingly disease-free survival benefits for patients of renal cell carcinoma from modern radical nephrectomy.[7,8] Robson's assertions significantly consolidated the position of radical nephrectomy as the principal treatment arm in the management algorithm of renal carcinoma. However, one cannot overlook the fact that most patients presented then harbored large, symptomatic, or locally advanced tumors requiring radical excision of the kidney with its coverings. Radical nephrectomy continued its primacy throughout the rest of the century.

The prevailing strident general espousal of radical nephrectomy did not altogether subvert the lingering interest in nephron-sparing surgery. Poutasse's improvization of the surgical technique of partial nephrectomy based on the segmental blood supply to the kidney and introduction of renal hypothermia, which forestalled ischemic damage, yielded more operative time, and permitted complex intrarenal surgery, in no uncertain terms, promoted nephron-sparing surgery and gained for it many converts.[9–11] Novick, Puigvert, Wickham, Marberger, and many others increasingly indulged in nephron-sparing surgery and consistently derived overall survival benefits akin to those in patients with disease of similar stage who underwent radical nephrectomy.[11–14] In 1975 Wickham reviewed the global literature (1954–1974) and reported a 5-year survival rate of 72% in 37 patients after partial nephrectomy for tumors in a solitary kidney or bilateral renal tumors.[14]

The 1980s undoubtedly constituted the watershed in nephron-sparing surgery. The advent of quality cross-sectional imaging and its liberal use identified an increasing number of small cortical tumors in otherwise healthy kidneys and most agreeably suited for nephron-sparing efforts. Similarly, proliferation of energy sources to achieve tissue cleavage as well as hemostasis provided the additional impetus for frequent performance of nephron-sparing surgery. Refinements in hypothermia and allied renoprotective measures in recent years have further facilitated complex intrarenal surgery. Renal hypothermia with ice slush is easily achievable and requires no sophisticated infrastructural support. In addition to surface hypothermia, there is an ever expanding list of pharmaceuticals which can be used selectively along with hypothermia to retard the adverse impact of renal ischemia, oxidative stress, and reperfusion injuries. These include among others vasoactive drugs, membrane-stabilizing drugs, calcium channel blockers, and catalytic antioxidants.

There are clear indications at present that minimally invasive approaches such as laparoscopic and robotic interventions will be increasingly used in this century and their impending ascendancy over open-nephron-sparing surgery will be aided and abetted by an impressive array of newly developed ablative technologies such as radiofrequency ablation (RFA), high-intensity focused ultrasound (HIFU), laser interstitial thermotherapy (LITT), microwave thermotherapy (MT), photon irradiation, and cryoablation.

REFERENCES

1. Harry WH. A history of partial nephrectomy for renal tumours. J Urol 2005; 173: 705.
2. Newman D. History of renal surgery. Lancet 1901; 23: 149.
3. Goldstein AE, Abeshouse BS. Partial resections of the kidney. A report of 6 cases and a review of the literature. J Urol 1939; 42: 15.
4. Vermooten V. Indications for conservative surgery in certain renal tumours: a study based on the growth pattern of the clear cell carcinoma. J Urol 1950; 64: 200.
5. Bell ET. A classification of renal tumours with observations on the frequency of the various types. J Urol 1938; 39: 238.
6. Semb C. Partial resection of the kidney: operative technique. Acta Chir Scand 1955; 109: 360.
7. Robson C. Radical nephrectomy for renal cell carcinoma. J Urol 1963; 89: 37.
8. Robson CJ, Churchill BM, Anderson W. The results of radical nephrectomy for renal cell carcinoma. J Urol 1969; 101: 297.
9. Poutasse EF. Partial nephrectomy: new techniques, approach, operative indication and review of 51 cases. J Urol 1962; 88: 153.
10. Wickham JEA, Hanley HF, Jockes AM, et al. Regional renal hypothermia. Br J Urol 1967; 39: 727.
11. Marberger M, Georgi M, Guenther R, et al. Simultaneous balloon occlusion of the renal artery and hypothermic perfusion in in situ surgery of the kidney. J Urol 1978; 119: 453.
12. Novick AC, Stewart BH, Straffon RA, et al. Partial nephrectomy in the treatment of renal adenocarcinoma. J Urol 1977; 118: 1977.
13. Puigvert A. Partial nephrectomy for renal tumour; 21 cases. Eur J Urol 1976; 2: 70.
14. Wickham JE. Conservative renal surgery for adenocarcinoma. The place of bench surgery. Br J Urol 1975; 47: 25.

2

Surgical anatomy of kidney relevant to nephron-sparing surgery

Arun Chawla and Larry W Belbeck

GROSS ANATOMY

The kidneys are paired solid organs that lie within the retroperitoneum on either side of the spine. The normal kidney in the adult male and female weighs approximately 150 g and 135 g, respectively. The dimensions of the kidney are related to the overall body size and the approximate measurements of a normal kidney are 10 to 12 cm in the cranial-caudial dimension, 5 to 7 cm in the medial-lateral dimension, and 3 cm in the anterior-posterior thickness.[1]

Kidneys are covered by a thin but tough fibro-elastic capsule, which strips easily from the parenchyma but can hold the sutures better than parenchyma. On the medial surface of either kidney is a depression, the renal hilum, which leads into the space called the 'renal sinus'. The urine-collecting structures and vessels occupy the renal sinus and exit the kidney through the hilum medially (Figure 2.1).

The adult kidney has a smooth convex lateral surface with rounded upper and lower poles. The renal parenchyma is divided into the outer cortex and inner medulla. The medulla consists of multiple distinct cortical segments, the renal 'pyramids'. The apex of each pyramid is the renal papilla, which points centrally into the renal sinus where it is cupped by an individual minor calyx of the collecting system. The number of pyramids corresponds to the number of minor calyces. Each kidney in its capsule is surrounded by a mass of adipose tissue called the perirenal fat, which is enclosed by the renal (Gerota's) fascia. This fascia is enclosed anteriorly and posteriorly by another layer of adipose tissue called the pararenal fat.

RELATIONS

The kidneys are remarkably mobile organs, and their positions vary with respiratory movements of the diaphragm as well as with changes in body posture.[2] The left kidney extends from the body of the 12th thoracic vertebra to the 3rd lumbar vertebra. The right kidney lies a little lower and usually extends from the top of the first lumbar vertebra to the bottom of the third lumbar vertebra. The kidneys lie on the psoas and the quadratus lumborum muscles (Figure 2.2).

The posterior surface of the right kidney is related to the 12th rib and the left to the 11th and 12th ribs. Although the posterior reflection of the pleura extends below the 12th rib, the lowermost lung edge lies above the 11th rib. The liver and the spleen are related posterolaterally to the suprahilar region of the kidney. The hepatic flexure of the colon lies anteriorly to the right kidney and the splenic flexure lies anterolateral to the left kidney (Figure 2.3).

RENAL VASCULATURE

The renal vessels enter the kidney via the renal hilum and from anteroposteriorly; the structures at the renal hilum are the renal vein, artery, and pelvis (Figure 2.4).

RENAL ARTERIES

The renal arteries lie at the level of the second lumbar vertebra below the origin of the superior mesenteric artery. The right renal artery often leaves the aorta at a

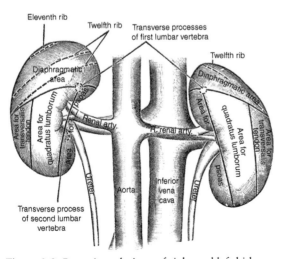

Figure 2.1 Demonstration of the renal vascular disposition in the cadaver and its relation to the collecting system after the removal of the anterior cortical layer of the left kidney. (1) Adrenal, (2) main renal artery, (3) major calyx, (4) renal papillae, (5) gonadal vein, (6) ureter. Reproduced from Rohen JW, Yokochi C, Lutjen-Drecol E. Color atlas of anatomy: a photographic study of the human body, 6th edition. With permission of Lippincott Wilkins.

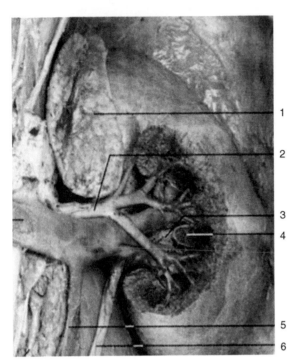

Figure 2.2 Posterior relations of right and left kidneys.

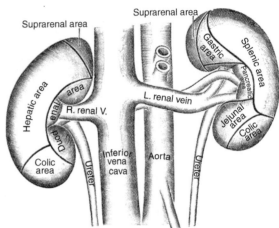

Figure 2.3 Anterior relations of right and left kidneys.

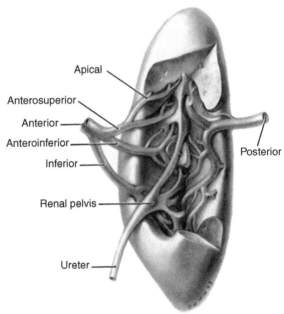

Figure 2.4 Medial view of the disposition of the renal vasculature and its relation to the collecting system at the renal hilum.

slightly higher level than the left and passes behind the inferior vena cava, hence it is longer than the left renal artery. The left renal artery lies horizontally.

The main renal artery divides into four or five segmental vessels. The first and the most constant segmental division is a posterior branch which arises from the main stem before it enters the renal hilum and proceeds posteriorly to the renal pelvis to supply a large posterior segment of the kidney (Figure 2.5). The remaining anterior division of the main renal artery branches as it enters the renal hilum. Four segmental branches originating from the anterior division are the apical, upper, middle, and lower segmental arteries. The segmental arteries course through the renal sinus and branch into the lobar arteries, which further divide and enter the parenchyma as interlobar arteries. These interlobar arteries course outwards between the pyramids and branch into arcuate arteries that give rise to multiple interlobular arteries.

The kidney has four constant vascular segments, which are termed apical, anterior, posterior, and basilar (lower) (Figure 2.6). The anterior segment is the largest and extends beyond the midplane of the kidney onto the posterior surface. A definite avascular plane exists at the junction of the anterior and posterior segments on the posterior surface of the kidney. The anatomic position of the vascular segments is constant. All segmental arteries are end arteries and ligation or injury to these vessels results in the loss of functioning renal parenchyma. Multiple renal arteries occur unilaterally in 25% and bilaterally in 10% of the population.[3]

VENOUS ANATOMY

The normal renal venous anatomy consists of two veins, right and left, terminating in the lateral aspect of the inferior vena cava (IVC). The left renal vein is longer and has thicker walls than the right renal vein. The left renal vein receives the gonadal vein inferiorly, left adrenal vein superiorly, and one or two large lumbar veins posteriorly. The right renal vein seldom drains a significant branch. The renal venous drainage system differs from

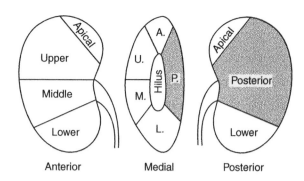

Figure 2.6 Vascular segments of the kidney in anterior, medial, and posterior views.

the arterial system in that the intrarenal venous system freely intercommunicates among various renal segments.

COLLECTING SYSTEM

The intrarenal collecting system consists of eight to ten minor calyces that ultimately drain into the renal pelvis. The anterior and posterior segments are drained by three calyces each, while the basilar and apical segments are drained by a single calyx each.

APPLIED ANATOMY IN RELATION TO NEPHRON-SPARING SURGERY

Nephron-sparing surgery is technically more challenging than *en bloc* removal of the kidney by radical nephrectomy and, therefore, it requires a better understanding of renal anatomy. Knowledge of the relationships of the tumor and its vascular supply to the collecting system and adjacent normal parenchyma is essential for preoperative assessment. Thus, more extensive and invasive preoperative imaging studies are sometimes necessary before nephron-sparing surgery.[4] These may include arteriography and occasionally venography. Arteriography may be done to delineate the intrarenal vasculature, which may aid in tumor excision while minimizing blood loss and injury to the normal adjacent parenchyma (Figure 2.7). It is most useful for non-peripheral tumors encompassing two or more renal arterial segments. Selective renal venography is performed in patients with large or centrally located tumors to evaluate intrarenal thrombosis and assess the adequacy of venous drainage of the planned renal remnant. Advances in helical computerized tomography (CT) and computer technology now allow the production of high-quality three-dimensional (3D) images of the renal vasculature and soft tissue

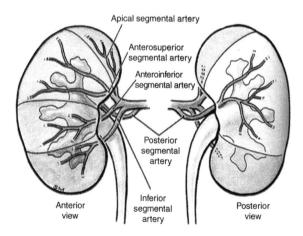

Figure 2.5 Renal artery and its principal divisions – anterior and posterior views.

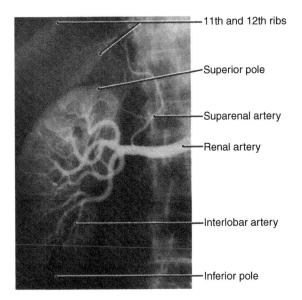

Figure 2.7 Angiographic depiction (anteroposterior) of the renal arterial system.

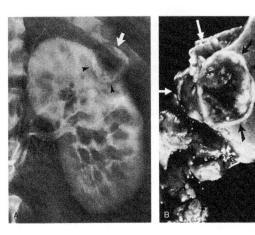

Figure 2.8 (A) Angiogram showing a peripheral tumor of the left kidney (black arrowheads and white arrow). (B) Resected specimen of the tumor (black arrows) along with peritumor envelopes (white arrows).

anatomy, and provide a topographic road map of the renal surface with multiplanar views of the intrarenal anatomy[5] (Figure 2.8).

ARTERIAL ANATOMY IN RELATION TO TUMOR LOCATION

Superior pole

In more than 75% of cases, the superior pole is related to three arteries which can be involved in nephron-sparing surgery:

1. The superior or apical segmental artery, which is not in close relation to the upper infundibulum and usually arises from the anterosuperior segmental artery.
2. Two other arteries, anterior and posterior, which are in close relationship to the upper infundibular surfaces, anteriorly and posteriorly.

Ligation of the superior (apical) segmental artery is easy, as its origin is quite proximal, and the artery related to the anterior surface of the upper infundibulum can also be ligated or coagulated without added care and any extra danger of extensive parenchymal injury. Management of the artery related to the posterior surface of the superior infundibulum is more complex, as risk of injury to this vessel during any partial nephrectomy

procedure is associated with significant hemorrhage and infarction of about 50% of the renal parenchyma.[6]

When the anterior and posterior surfaces of the superior pole are supplied only by the polar superior artery, nephron-sparing surgery is relatively easy, because its ligation results in a clean line of demarcation making resection of the superior polar tumors a more comfortable exercise.[6] The peripheral tumors are associated with splaying of the surrounding vessels and resection of these tumors can be achieved by careful ligation of the vessels around the tumors (Figure 2.9).

Inferior pole

In two-thirds of patients, the lower pole of the kidney is supplied by the inferior segmental branch of the anterior division of the main renal artery. This courses in front of the ureteropelvic junction and, on entering the inferior pole, divides into two branches supplying the anterior and posterior surfaces. In the rest of the cases, the lower pole is supplied jointly by two arteries, a branch from the inferior segmental artery anteriorly and another from the inferior branch of the posterior segmental artery posteriorly. Ligation of both these branches during partial nephrectomy involving the lower pole tumors does not result in ischemia of the remaining parenchyma.

Midzone

The midzone is mainly supplied by the anterior division of the renal artery. Nephron-sparing surgery of the midzone involves infringement of the calyceal anatomy. In two-thirds of the cases, the middle group of calyces

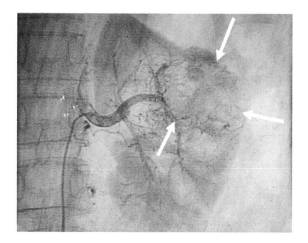

Figure 2.9 Angiogram showing a peripheral tumor in the left kidney (arrows) splaying the divisions of the anteriosuperior segmental artery.

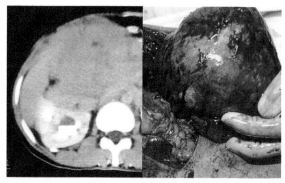

Figure 2.10 CT scan and operative photograph demonstrating a large central tumor of the right kidney.

is associated with the superior and/or inferior calyceal groups and hence resection in this region should preserve adequate calyceal drainage to the remaining poles. Careful closure of calyceal ends after resection is essential to avoid postoperative urinary fistula or collection (see Chapter 11 Controversies in nephron-sparing surgery). In a third of cases, midzone calyceal drainage is independent of the superior or inferior calyceal groups and, in these cases, resection of the midzone does not present additional difficulties.

Midzone tumors involve resection of the central position of the kidney while maintaining the blood supply to the remaining renal parenchyma at the poles. Technically, it is more challenging than polar nephron-sparing resections and always requires a preoperative selective renal angiogram to determine the exact intrarenal arterial anatomy and to ascertain the resectability of the lesion. Centrally-placed tumors need meticulous dissection of the arteries supplying the tumor under hypothermic and avascular control. Normal restoration of renal configuration and function can be maintained after complete resection (Figures 2.10 and 2.11).

Dorsal kidney

The posterior or dorsal part of the kidney is supplied by the posterior segmental artery, which is the first division of the main renal artery. This divides into three constant subdivisions – superior, middle and inferior, supplying the respective areas of the dorsal kidney. The middle branch sometimes interdigitates with the anterior branches supplying the midportion of the

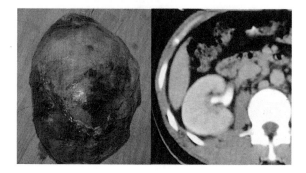

Figure 2.11 Excised specimen of the tumor (from Figure 2.10) and postoperative CT scan demonstrating the reconfigured functioning kidney.

kidney. Resection of midzone tumors requires the identification and ligation of anterior branches related to the midkidney and middle subdivision of the posterior segmental artery. The tumors arising close to the hilum need careful isolation of the principal renal vessels and the renal pelvis with the upper ureter (Figure 2.12). Preliminary access to vessels is mandatory and the renal pedicle must be completely exposed and skeletonized, as midzone tumors sometimes receive secondary branches from arteries of other segments.[7] Resection of tumors in this zone is always performed under hypothermic and ischemic control.

VENOUS ANATOMY

Although the intrarenal veins have no segmental organization, in the majority of the cases two or three major

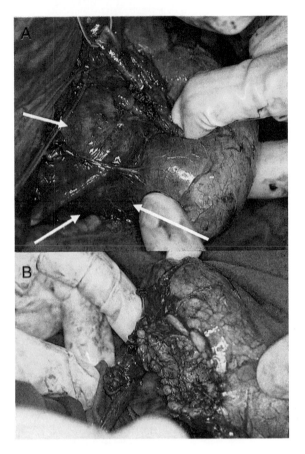

Figure 2.12 (A) Hilar renal tumor (white arrows) after mobilization of the main renal artery, vein, and renal pelvis. (B) Normal restoration of renal configuration after the resection.

CONCLUSIONS

Various surgical techniques are available for performing partial nephrectomy for solid renal lesions. The spectrum of surgical options includes tumor enucleation, polar segmental nephrectomy with preliminary ligation of the appropriate renal arterial branch, wedge resection, major transverse resection, and extracorporeal partial nephrectomy with autotransplantation (see Chapter 11). In the majority of patients undergoing conservative sugery for renal cell carcinoma, excision is performed by wedge or segmental resection obtaining a thin margin of adjacent normal parenchyma. Preoperative imaging studies are essential to know the arterial anatomy in relation to the tumor location. Extracorporeal nephron-sparing surgery with autotransplantation is indicated only in rare cases with exceptionally large tumors and anatomically challenging tumors. The basic principles of all these nephron-sparing surgical techniques include early vascular control, avoidance of renal ischemia, precise control of the collecting system, careful hemostasis, and closure of the renal defect.[8]

REFERENCES

1. Anderson JK, Kabalin JN, Cadeddu JA. Surgical anatomy of the retroperitoneum, adrenals, kidneys and ureters. In: Kavoussi LR, Novick AC, Partin AW, Peters CA, Wein AJ (eds) Campbell-Walsh Urology, 9th edn. Philadelphia: Saunders, 2007.
2. Gosling JA, Dixon JS, Humpherson JR. Gross anatomy of the kidneys and upper urinary tract. In: Gosling JA, Dixon JS, Humpherson JR, eds. Functional Anatomy of the Urinary Tract. An Integrated Text and Colour Atlas. London: Churchill Livingstone, 1983: 1–40.
3. Novick AC. Open surgery of the kidney. In: Kavoussi LR, Novick AC, Partin AW, Peters CA, Wein AJ (eds) Campbell-Walsh Urology, 9th edn. Philadelphia: Saunders, 2007.
4. Uzzo RG, Novick AC. Nephron sparing surgery for renal tumours: indications, techniques and outcomes. J Urol 2001; 166: 6–18.
5. Coll DM, Uzzo TG, Herts BR, et al. 3-Dimensional volume rendered computerized tomography for preoperative evaluation and intraoperative treatment of patients undergoing nepron sparing surgery. J Urol 1999; 161: 1097.
6. Sampaio FJB. Anatomic background for nephron sparing surgery in renal cell carcinoma. J Urol 1992; 147: 999–1005.
7. Sampaio FJB, Schiavini JL, Favorito LA. Proportional analysis of the arterial segments. Urol Res 1993; 21: 371–4.
8. Novick AC. Partial nephrectomy for renal cell carcinoma. Urol Clin North Am 1987; 14: 419.

trunks join to form the main renal vein. During partial nephrectomy, ligature of many tributaries of major trunks can be done, enabling ample exposure of the intrarenal branches of the main renal artery that usually lie in a deep plane within the renal hilum. In the presence of abundant venous collaterals, ligation of the major venous trunk is not associated with any infarction or loss of functioning of the renal parenchyma.

3

Pathology of renal cell carcinoma

Saleh Binsaleh, Kathy Chorneyko, Arun Chawla, and Anil Kapoor

INTRODUCTION

Renal cell carcinoma (RCC) was originally named *hypernephroma* due to its histologic resemblance to the adrenal gland. In 1960, Oberling et al[1] demonstrated its origin from the proximal renal tubule based on the ultrastructural features. The tumor was then renamed *renal cell adenocarcinoma* or *renal cell carcinoma*.

RCC is the most commonly diagnosed renal malignancy, accounting for 85% of all renal cancers, with about 23 000 new cases and 8000 new deaths from kidney cancer reported in the United States every year.[2] This incidence appears to be increasing and in 2007 it is estimated that around 51 000 new cases will be diagnosed with renal malignancy in the United States alone.[3]

RCC has a 1.6:1.0 male predominance, with a peak incidence in the sixth and seventh decades, although patients in the first two decades of life have been reported.

The most consistent risk factors include obesity (particularly in women), smoking, hypertension, acquired renal cystic disease associated with endstage renal failure, and a family history of RCC.[4] About 2% of renal cancer is associated with inherited syndromes (Table 3.1).

Clinical presentation varies from hematuria, flank pain, or a palpable mass to incidentally detected tumors by imaging techniques done for other reasons. In some instances, systemic symptoms (paraneoplastic syndrome) or symptoms of metastasis can be the only presenting features.

In this chapter the most recent WHO classification for renal cell carcinoma will be outlined. This will include a description of the pertinent immunohistochemical and genetic features from a clinical standpoint (Table 3.2).

STAGING SYSTEM FOR RENAL CELL CARCINOMA

The staging system for RCC, recommended by the American Joint Committee on Cancer (AJCC), is shown in Table 3.3. The latest edition (2002) incorporates tumor size, extent of local invasion, involvement of large veins, adrenal gland, or lymph nodes, and distant metastasis. Prognosis is closely related to the stage of the disease.[5]

INTEGRATED STAGING ALGORITHMS

The TNM staging system (Table 3.3) is currently the most extensively used system for RCC. However, new comprehensive staging modalities have emerged in an attempt to improve prognostication by combining other pathologic and clinical variables. Tumor stage, tumor grade, and Eastern Cooperative Oncology Group (ECOG) patient performance status (PS) remain the most useful clinically available predictors of patient outcome for RCC. Additionally, several other clinical and pathologic characteristics have been identified as having an impact on the clinical behavior and subsequent survival in patients with localized and advanced RCC.[6]

The University of California–Los Angeles Integrated Staging System (UISS) was developed to better stratify patients into prognostic categories using statistical tools that accurately define the probability of survival of an individual patient.[7] The initial UISS contained five groups based on TNM stage, Fuhrman nuclear grade, and Eastern Cooperative Oncology Group performance status. For patients in UISS groups I to V, the projected 2- and 5-year survival rates are 96% and 94% (group I), 89% and 67% (group II), 66% and 39% (group III), 42% and 23% (group IV), and 9% and 0% (group V). The UISS was internally validated using a bootstrapping technique and then using an expanded database of patients treated at University of California– Los Angeles (UCLA) between 1989 and 2000,[8] with external data from 576 RCC patients treated at MD Anderson Cancer Center and in Nijmegen, the Netherlands,[9,10] and most recently with 4202 RCC patients from eight international centers.[11]

Table 3.1 Familial renal cell carcinoma: syndromic and non-syndromic presentation

Syndrome	Gene	Tumor
VHL	VHL (3p25)	Clear cell RCC, renal cysts, retinal and CNS hemangioblastomas, pheochromocytomas, pancreatic cysts and neuroendocrine tumors, endolymphatic sac tumors, epididymal and broad ligament cystadenomas
Tuberous sclerosis	TSC1, TSC2	Angiomyolipoma, clear cell, ependymal nodules, adenoma sebaceum, subungual fibromas, retinal hamartomas
Constitutional chromosome 3 translocation	Responsible gene not found. VHL gene mutated in some families	Clear cell
Familial renal carcinoma	Gene not identified	Clear cell
Hereditary PRCC	c-MET	Papillary type 1
BHD	BHD	Chromophobe, renal oncocytomas, hybrid oncocytic and clear cell carcinomas, lung cysts, spontaneous pneumothorax
Familial oncocytoma	Partial or complete loss of multiple chromosomes	Oncocytoma
Hereditary leiomyoma–RCC	FH	Papillary type 2, uterine leiomyomas and leiomyosarcomas, cutaneous nodules (leiomyomas)

BHD, Birt–Hogg–Dubé; RCC, renal cell carcinoma; VHL, Von Hippel–Lindau; FH; fumarate hydratase.

The UISS has been subsequently modified into a simplified system, based on separate stratification of patients with metastatic and non-metastatic disease into low-risk, intermediate-risk, and high-risk groups.[12] This provides a clinically useful system for predicting postoperative outcome and a unique tool for risk assignment and outcome analysis to help determine follow-up regimens and eligibility for clinical trials. The incorporation of molecular tumor markers (discussed later) into future staging systems is expected to revolutionize the approach to diagnosis and prognosis of cancer.[13]

CLASSIFICATION OF RENAL CELL CARCINOMA

The most accepted classification system for RCC originated from a consensus conference in Rochester, Minnesota, in 1997 and was subsequently modified in the 2004 WHO (World Health Organization) classification.[14] This classification system (Table 3.4) will be used for the purpose of discussion in the following sections:

- Clear cell RCC
- Multilocular clear cell RCC
- Papillary RCC
- Chromophobe RCC
- Collecting duct RCC
- Renal medullary carcinoma
- Xp11 translocation carcinomas
- Carcinoma associated with neuroblastoma
- Mucinous tubular and spindle cell carcinoma
- RCC unclassified

Familial renal cancer

Inherited or familial predisposition to renal neoplasia is present in 2–3% of renal tumors. Table 3.1 lists known

Table 3.2 Main pathologic and genetic features of adult renal cell carcinoma according to the 2004 WHO classification[14]

RCC subtype	Incidence	Development	Cell/tissue characteristics	Growth pattern	Prognosis	Genetic abnormality
Clear cell	75%	Solitary, rare multicentric or bilateral	Clear cytoplasm; cells with eosinophilic cytoplasm occasionally	Solid, tubular, cystic, rare papillae	Aggressiveness according to grade, stage and sarcomatoid change	$-3p$, $+5q22$, $-6q$, $-8p$, $-9p$, $-14q$
Multilocular cystic	Rare	Solitary, rare bilateral	Clear cytoplasm, small dark nuclei	Cystic, no solid component	No progression or metastases	VHL gene mutation
Papillary	10%	Multicentric, bilateral or solitary	Type 1 (basophilic) or type 2 (eosinophilic)	Tubulopapillary, solid	Aggressiveness according to grade, stage, and sarcomatoid change	$+3q$, $+7$, $+8$, $+12$, $+16$, $+17$, $+20$, $-Y$
Chromophobe	5%	Solitary	Pale or eosinophilic granular cytoplasm	Solid	10% mortality	-1, -2, -6, -10, -17, -21, hypodiploidy
Collecting ducts of Bellini	1%	Solitary	Eosinophilic cytoplasm	Irregular channels	Aggressive, 2/3 of patients die within 2 years	$-1q$, $-6p$, $-8p$, $-13q$, $-21q$, $-3p$ (rare)
Medullary	Rare	Solitary	Eosinophilic cytoplasm	Reticular pattern	Mean survival of 15 weeks after diagnosis	Unknown

(Continued)

Table 3.2 (Continued)

RCC subtype	Incidence	Development	Cell/tissue characteristics	Growth pattern	Prognosis	Genetic abnormality
Xp11 translocation	Rare	Solitary	Clear and eosinophilic cells	Tubulopapillary	Indolent	t (X; 1) (p11.2; q21), t (X; 17) (p11.2; q25), other
After neuroblastoma	Rare	Solitary	Eosinophilic cells with oncocytoid features	Solid	Related to grade and stage	Allelic imbalance at 20q13
Mucinous tubular and spindle cell	Rare	Solitary	Tubules, extracellular mucin, and spindle cells	Solid	Rare metastases,	-1, -4, -6, -8, -13, -14, $+7$, $+11$, $+16$, $+17$
Unclassified	4% to 6%	Solitary	Variable, sarcomatoid	Solid	High mortality	Unknown

Table 3.3 TNM staging system for renal cell carcinoma

		Definition of AJCC TNM Stage for Renal Cell Cancer*
Primary tumor (T)		
TX		Primary tumor cannot be assessed
T0		No evidence of primary tumor
T1		Tumor less than 7 cm in diameter and limited to the kidney
	T1a	Tumor 4 cm or less in greatest dimension and limited to kidney
	T1b	Tumor more than 4 cm but less than 7 cm, and limited to kidney
T2		Tumor more than 7 cm in greatest dimension limited to the kidney
T3		Tumor extends into major veins or invades the adrenal gland or perinephric tissues, but not beyond Gerota's fascia
	T3a	Tumor directly invades the adrenal gland or perinephric tissues but not beyond Gerota's fascia
	T3b	Tumor grossly extends into the renal vein or its segmental (muscle-containing) branches, or vena cava below the diaphragm
	T3c	Tumor grossly extends into the vena cava above the diaphragm or invades the wall of the vena cava
T4		Tumor invades beyond Gerota's fascia
Regional lymph nodes (N)†		
NX	Regional lymph nodes cannot be assessed	
N0	No regional lymph node metastases	
N1	Metastasis in a single regional lymph node	
N2	Metastases in more than one regional lymph node	
Distant metastasis (M)		
MX	Distant metastasis cannot be assessed	
M0	No distant metastasis	
M1	Distant metastasis	

*Used with the permission of the American Joint Committee on Cancer (AJCC), Chicago, Illinois. The original source for this
  material is the AJCC Cancer Staging Manual, Sixth Edition (2002) published by Springer-Verlag New York,
  www.springeronline.com.
†Laterality does not affect the N classification.

inherited syndromes that predispose to renal tumors as presented in the 2004 WHO classification.[14] Each of these syndromes is associated with a distinct histologic type of renal cell carcinoma or other kidney tumor.

From the clinical point of view, hereditary renal cancers show a tendency to be multiple and bilateral, may have a family history, and present at an earlier age than the non-familial and non-hereditary renal neoplasms.[15]

Clear cell (conventional) renal cell carcinoma

This type of RCC accounts for about 75% of surgically removed renal cancer.[16] According to the 2004 WHO classification, all kidney tumors of clear cell type of any size are considered malignant.[14] These tumors can be as small as 1 cm or less and discovered incidentally, or they can be bulky and weigh several kilograms. The majority are sporadic, but familial forms are also recognized, including Von Hippel–Lindau disease, tuberous sclerosis, and familial clear cell renal cancer (Table 3.1), 0.5–3.0% of patients have bilateral disease and 4–13% have multiple ipsilateral tumors.[1,16] This tumor is believed to arise from the proximal tubular epithelium, and cytogenetically is associated with inactivation of a tumor suppressor gene on chromosome 3p. The term 'granular cell' indicates RCC with acidophilic cytoplasm, a specific tumor category in the 1998 WHO classification; however, tumors with this morphology

Table 3.4 WHO classification of kidney tumors[14]		
Familial renal cancer		
Renal cell tumors		
Malignant	Benign	
Clear cell renal cell carcinoma	Papillary adenoma	
Multilocular clear cell renal cell carcinoma	Oncocytoma	
Papillary renal cell carcinoma		
Chromophobe renal cell carcinoma		
Carcinoma of the collecting ducts of Bellini		
Renal medullary carcinoma		
Xp11 translocation carcinomas		
Carcinoma associated with neuroblastoma		
Mucinous tubular and spindle cell carcinoma		
Renal cell carcinoma unclassified		
Metanephric tumors		
Metanephric adenoma		
Metanephric adenofibroma		
Metanephric stromal tumors		
Mixed mesenchymal and epithelial tumors		
Cystic nephroma		
Mixed epithelial and stromal tumor		
Synovial sarcoma		
Nephroblastic tumors		
Nephrogenic rests		
Nephroblastoma		
Cystic partially differentiated nephroblastoma		
Neuroendocrine tumors		
Carcinoid		
Neuroendocrine carcinoma		
Primitive neuroectodermal tumor		
Neuroblastoma		
Pheochromocytoma		
Other tumors		
Mesenchymal tumors		
Hematopoietic and lymphoid tumors		
Germ cell tumors		
Metastatic tumors		

are now included among the clear cell type based on the absence of genetic and clinical differences between the two morphologic types.[17]

Grossly, clear RCC is classically solitary, well circumscribed, solid, variegated, and orange to yellow in color. Areas of necrosis, hemorrhage, and fibrosis can be observed. The tumor can infiltrate adjacent parenchyma, and may extend into the renal vein. Cysts are commonly present and vary in size (Figure 3.1).

Under microscopy (Figure 3.2), clear RCC is composed of cells with abundant clear to pale cytoplasm (hence the name). The cytoplasm is rich in lipids and glycogen,

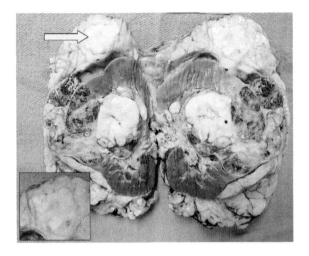

Figure 3.1 Clear cell renal cell carcinoma. This tumor shows a variegated, heterogeneous appearance with extension into the perinephric fat (arrow and inset).

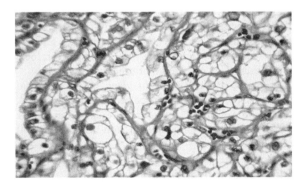

Figure 3.2 Clear cell renal cell carcinoma. Tubular structures are lined by clear cells and separated by a delicate capillary network.

which dissolve during processing and provide the characteristic clear cytoplasm. Tumor cells form compact nests, tubules, or cystic structures in a rich prominent network of thin-walled blood vessels (sinusoidal vasculature). Tubules and microcysts are usually filled with red blood cells or proteinaceous fluid. Tumor cell nuclei show variation in size, shape, and degree of nucleolar prominence, these features forming the basis of the *Fuhrman nuclear grading system*:[18]

Grade 1: small round uniform nuclei, up to 10 μm, inconspicuous nucleoli.
Grade 2: nuclei slightly irregular, up to 15 μm, and uniform nucleoli.
Grade 3: very irregular nuclei, up to 20 μm, and large prominent nucleoli.
Grade 4: bizarre shape nuclei, spindle or multilobated, more than 20 μm, macronucleoli (Figure 3.3).

Mitotic activity is not considered as a component of grading as it varies among tumors and does not correlate well with prognosis.[17] When tumor heterogeneity is present, the overall grade is based on the highest grade area. The survival rates at 5 years are 67% for grade 1 tumors, 56% for grade 2 tumors, 33% for grade 3 tumors, and 8% for grade 4 tumors.[17]

A variant of this neoplasm is *multilocular cystic clear cell RCC*. This type is considered a separate entity according to the latest 2004 WHO classification.[14] There is a male predominance of 3:1, with age ranging from 20 to 76 years. This tumor is composed entirely of cysts with no solid component. The cyst wall is lined by clear cells which form small aggregates in the septa between the cysts. Cases with expansive nodules are excluded. This tumor variant is usually low grade with an excellent prognosis and no cases of malignant behavior have been reported.[16]

A *sarcomatoid* component can be associated with any type of RCC, but occasionally RCC is entirely sarcomatoid, with no recognizable epithelial elements (Figure 3.4).

Clear cell RCC must be differentiated from other malignant tumors and non-neoplastic conditions. Xanthogranulomatous pyelonephritis, which is usually associated with a calculus or calculi, is the most important

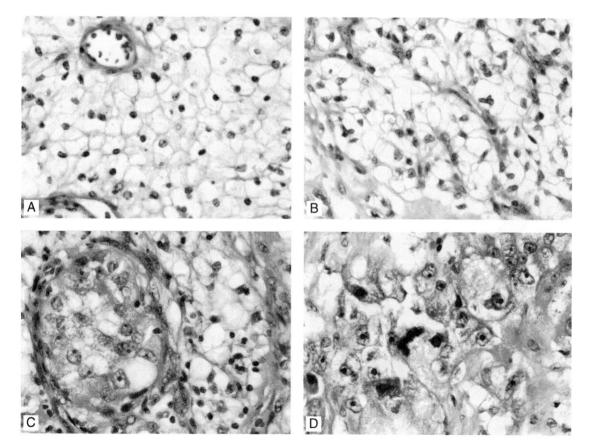

Figure 3.3 Clear cell renal cell carcinoma Fuhrman nuclear grade 1, 2, 3, and 4 (A, B, C, and D, respectively).

benign condition that can be grossly and microscopically mistaken as clear cell RCC. The inflammatory cell infiltrate contains numerous histiocytes that may be misinterpreted as tumor cells; however, the vascular stroma characteristic of clear cell RCC is absent.[16] The cytoplasm of the histiocytes can be clear but is also foamy. The histiocytes are typically admixed with other inflammatory cells such as lymphocytes and plasma cells (Figure 3.5). Malacoplakia is another inflammatory process usually associated with immunosuppression, which may resemble clear cell RCC. Its gross appearance, characterized by tan-brown masses infiltrating the perinephric fat, might be highly suggestive of RCC. Histologically, the inflammatory cell infiltrate is predominantly composed of esinophilic histiocytes, resembling the granular cells of clear cell RCC. However, extensive histologic sampling fails to identify the characteristic histologic features of clear cell RCC.[17] Also, in malacoplakia, Michaelis–Gutmann laminated bodies are seen in the cytoplasm of some histiocytes, assuring the correct diagnosis.

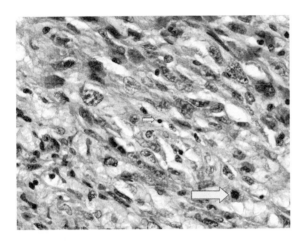

Figure 3.4 Renal cell carcinoma, sarcomatoid features. Elongated, spindled malignant cells are present with interspersed small lymphocytes (small arrow). One mitotic figure is present (large arrow).

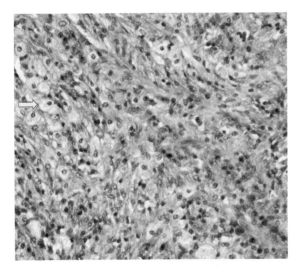

Figure 3.5 Xanthogranulomatous pyelonephritis. Mixed inflammatory infiltrate composed of lymphocytes, plasma cells, and foamy histiocytes (arrow).

Papillary renal cell carcinoma

This tumor has been previously referred to as chromophil renal cell carcinoma. It was initially described in 1989 and it accounts for 10–15% of RCC. There is a 5:1 male predominance, a better prognosis, and a lower metastatic potential compared to other types of RCC.[17,19] The 5-year survival is estimated to be 90% for sporadic papillary RCC. This tumor is believed to arise from the proximal tubular epithelium and cytogenetically is associated with trisomy or tetrasomy of chromosomes 7 and 17 and loss of chromosome Y.[20,21] The risk of papillary RCC increases in patients with endstage renal failure who are on dialysis (discussed later).

There are two subtypes of papillary renal cell carcinoma.[14,15] *Type 1* tumors are papillary lesions covered by small basophilic cells with pale cytoplasm and small oval nuclei with indistinct nucleoli (Figure 3.6) and *type 2* tumors are papillary lesions covered by large cells with abundant eosinophilic cytoplasm. Type 2 cells are typified by pseudostratification and large, spherical nuclei with distinct nucleoli. Type 2 tumors are genetically more heterogeneous, have a poorer prognosis, and may arise from type 1 tumors.

Grossly, papillary RCC is usually friable, multifocal, pseudoencapsulated, and spherical and may be light gray, tan, yellow, or brown (Figure 3.7). Some tumors have extensive necrosis and hemorrhage. Calcification and cystic degeneration are common.

Microscopically, it appears as papillary or tubulopapillary structures lined by a single layer of tumor cells. The stroma of the fibrovascular cores contains abundant foamy macrophages, and calcified 'psammoma bodies' may be present. Papillary RCC sometimes has a sarcomatoid component, but less commonly than with clear cell RCC.[22,23]

The same grading system proposed for clear cell RCC may be used for papillary RCC;[17] however, its prognostic significance is not as well established as in clear cell RCC.

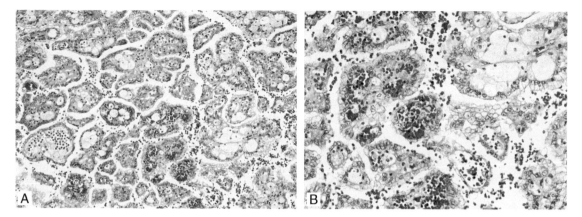

Figure 3.6 Papillary renal cell carcinoma type 1. (A) Low-power image showing numerous papillary structures. (B) Higher-power image of the papillae with fibrovascular cores focally containing foamy histiocytes.

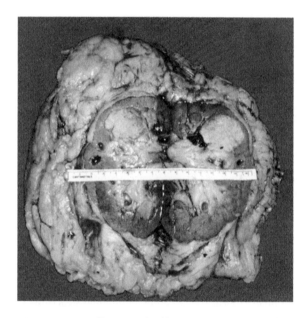

Figure 3.7 Papillary renal cell carcinoma with a homogeneous yellow/tan color.

Chromophobe renal cell carcinoma

Chromophobe RCC was discovered by Bannasch in 1974 while conducting experiments of renal cancer induction in rats, and was first described in humans in 1985 by Thoenes.[17,24] This tumor accounts for about 5% of RCC and has equal sex distribution. It carries a better prognosis than clear RCC with an estimated 5-year survival of 78%.[25]

This tumor is believed to arise from intercalated cells in the distal collecting tubule, and cytogenetically it is characterized by the loss of entire chromosomes (1, 2, 6, 10, 13, 17, and 21).[26]

The Birt–Hogg–Dubé syndrome is a rare autosomal dominant disorder characterized by hair follicle hamartomas (fibrofolliculomas) of the face and neck. About 15% of affected patients have multiple renal tumors, most often chromophobe or mixed chromophobe–oncocytomas. Occasionally, papillary or clear cell renal cell carcinoma develops in patients with this syndrome.[27]

Grossly, the tumor is usually solitary, spherical, solid, and well circumscribed. It has a brownish or gray cut surface. Hemorrhage and necrosis are usually absent or minimal.

Microscopically, the tumor cells are arranged in sheets intersected by thick fibrovascular strands. Two distinct cell types have been identified for this tumor: *typical* and *eosinophilic*. The typical variant is composed of large, polygonal cells of variable size, prominent thick cell membranes (plant-like), and pale or finely granular cytoplasm (Figure 3.8). The esinophilic type is characterized by prominent tubular architecture, cells containing dense granular cytoplasm, and pronounced eosinophilia. A 'perinuclear halo' is a characteristic feature due to cytoplasmic retraction away from the nucleus.[28,29] The nuclei are often irregular with a 'raisinoid' appearance (Figure 3.9).

These features of the eosinophilic variant of chromophobe RCC may make it difficult to distinguish from oncocytoma. Compared to oncocytoma, chromophobe RCC has a positive immunohistochemical staining for the epithelial membrane antigen and parvalbumin, but no reaction to vimentin. Hale's colloidal iron histochemical

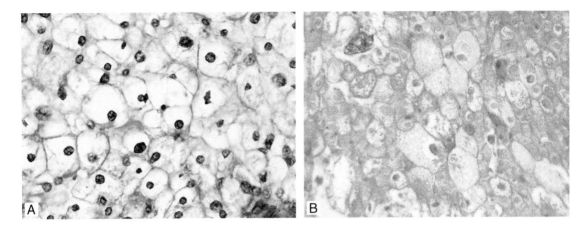

Figure 3.8 (A) Classical chromophobe renal cell carcinoma. (B) Positive Hale's colloidal iron reaction.

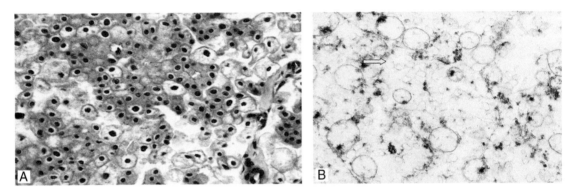

Figure 3.9 (A) Eosinophilic variant of chromophobe renal cell carcinoma. (B) Electron microscopy of chromophobe renal cell carcinoma showing numerous cytoplasmic vesicles (arrow).

staining is positive. Under electron microscopy oncocytoma has numerous cytoplasmic mitochondria while chromophobe RCC has numerous cytoplasmic membrane-bound vesicles.[26] Their origin is unknown but their formation may be related to mitochondria (Figure 3.10).

Collecting duct carcinoma

Also called Bellini's duct carcinoma, this tumor accounts for about 1% of surgically resected carcinomas of the kidney.[14,30] It carries a poor prognosis as the stage is often advanced at the time of diagnosis. The mean patient age is 55 years, with a slight male predominance.[14] This tumor arises from the collecting duct epithelium and cytogenetically it is associated with loss of heterozygosity in chromosomes 1q and 6p.[31]

Grossly, the tumor cut surface is gray-white. It has indistinct borders, an epicenter in the medulla, central necrosis, and it often invades into the perirenal tissues.

Microscopically, the tumor cells are composed of cuboidal and columnar cells with hyperchromatic and pleomorphic nuclei (Figure 3.11). The cells can form tubules, ducts, nests, or cords, and can display a 'hobnail' appearance when lining luminal structures.[30] The stroma commonly appears with a prominent desmoplastic and inflammatory response around the tumor. The immunophenotype has been expanded in the 2004 WHO classification:[14] it is positive for keratins of low (LMW) and high molecular weight (HMW) and vimentin, but molecular alterations are poorly understood. A sarcomatoid component can be seen in 30% of cases and is associated with the poor prognosis.

A variant of this neoplasm has been designated *low-grade collecting duct carcinoma*, often cystic with similar microscopic findings to classic collecting duct carcinoma. It does not infiltrate the adjacent normal parenchyma, or feature the desmoplastic and inflammatory reaction

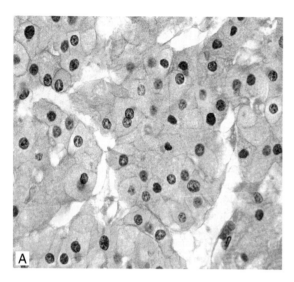 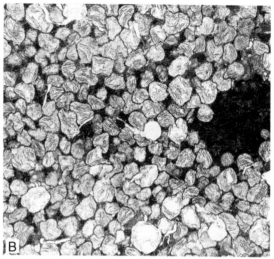

Figure 3.10 Oncocytoma differs from the eosinophilic variant of chromophobe renal cell carcinoma by the presence of numerous mitochondria in the cytoplasm of the tumor cells. (A) Small sheets and cords of uniform eosinophilic cells. (B) Electron microscopy showing abundant mitochondria in the cytoplasm.

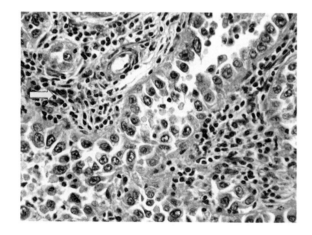

Figure 3.11 Collecting duct carcinoma showing tubules lined by columnar and cuboidal cells. There is a prominent inflammatory response around the tumor cells (arrow).

seen in the classic form. This variant has a low nuclear grade and stage, and prognosis is favorable.[16]

The main differential diagnosis of collecting duct carcinoma includes a high-grade RCC or urothelial carcinoma with glandular differentiation. Upper tract imaging often suggests urothelial carcinoma and patients may have positive urine cytology.[14,32,33]

Renal medullary carcinoma

This type affects young people with sickle cell disease or trait. Davis et al[34] initially described it in 1995 in a series of 33 patients, all of whom were African Americans. It usually presents at an advanced stage and carries a dismal prognosis.[14]

It is hypothesized that medullary carcinoma arises from the terminal collecting ducts and their adjacent papillary epithelium, which, in sickle cell disorders, seem to undergo abnormal proliferation. It is thought that this proliferation consists of transitional cells rather than columnar cells.

Grossly, the tumor is poorly circumscribed and occupies primarily the renal medulla with invasion of the renal calyces; satellite lesions are often present on the renal cortex.

Microscopically, the tumor usually demonstrates a distinctive reticular growth pattern reminiscent of yolk sac testicular tumors of the reticular type with some transitions to a more adenoid cystic appearance. The tumor cells are dark staining with large pale nuclei and prominent nucleoli. Acute inflammation and stromal proliferation are often present and lymphatic and/or vascular invasion are usually seen at the time of resection.

The immunohistochemical profile of renal medullary carcinoma has not been consistent in the reported cases. Keratin positivity has been reported in most cases, with diffuse positivity for vimentin and sometimes positivity for epithelial membrane antigen and carcinoembryonic antigen. Luminal mucin and sometimes the stroma has been noted to stain positively for lectin and mucicarmine in a number of cases. The overlap of the immunohistochemical features of renal medullary carcinoma with collecting duct carcinoma and urothelial carcinoma nullifies the diagnostic utility of immunohistochemical agents. The histologic resemblance and overlapping immunohistochemistry between this tumor and collecting duct carcinoma may raise the argument that this is a spectrum of the same neoplasm presenting in distinct clinical settings.

Renal carcinoma associated with Xp11.2 translocation/TFE3 gene fusions

This is a new entity added to the 2004 WHO classification of renal cell tumors.[14] This type of RCC is defined by different translocations involving chromosome Xp11.2, all resulting in gene fusions involving the TFE3 gene.[35] This carcinoma predominantly affects children and young adults. The ASPL-TFE3 translocation carcinomas characteristically present at an advanced stage associated with lymph node metastases. RCC associated with Xp11.2 translocations resembles clear cell RCC on gross examination and seems to have an indolent evolution, even with metastasis. The histopathologic appearance is that of a papillary carcinoma with clear cells and cells with granular eosinophilic cytoplasm. These cells display nuclear immunoreactivity for TFE3 protein.[35]

Renal cell carcinoma associated with neuroblastoma

A few cases of RCC arise in long-term survivors of childhood neuroblastoma. Males and females are equally affected with a mean age of 13.5 years, and can be unilateral or bilateral. This tumor entity is heterogeneous, shows oncocytoid features, and was not recognized in the previous WHO classification.[14,36] Allelic imbalances occur at the 20q13 locus. The prognosis is similar to other RCCs.

Mucinous, tubular, and spindle cell carcinoma

This entity, included for the first time in the 2004 WHO classification of renal tumors,[14] carries a female predominance and the mean age of 53 years. It presents as a circumscribed asymptomatic mass on ultrasound examination. Metastases have been rarely reported. This tumor is a low-grade carcinoma composed of tightly packed tubules separated by pale mucinous stroma and a spindle cell component (Figure 3.12). It seems to derive from the distal nephron. It has a combination of losses involving chromosomes 1, 4, 6, 8, 13, and 14, and gains of chromosomes 7, 11, 16, and 17.[37]

Renal cell carcinoma, unclassified

This comprises the remaining 4–5% of surgically resected renal carcinomas that show architectural and/or cytologic features that do not fit any type of RCC described above.[14] Included under this category is the RCC with pure sarcomatoid morphology.

Features which might place a carcinoma in this category include: (1) composites of recognized types, (2) pure sarcomatoid morphology without recognizable epithelial elements, (3) mucin production, (4) rare mixtures of epithelial and stromal elements, and (5) unrecognizable cell types.[38]

Sarcomatoid change may be seen in all types of RCC with no evidence to suggest that RCC develops 'de novo' as sarcomatoid carcinoma, therefore the 2004 WHO classification in contrast to the previous WHO classification does not consider it as an entity but rather as a progression of any RCC. Sarcomatoid carcinoma appears grossly as a pale fleshy mass, and histologically is composed of malignant spindle cells with focal areas of the underlying renal cell carcinoma (Figure 3.4).

RENAL CELL CARCINOMA ASSOCIATED WITH ACQUIRED CYSTIC DISEASE OF THE KIDNEY

This entity is discussed here for the purpose of completion of all the different pathologic appearances of RCCs.

Acquired cystic disease of the kidney (ACDK) is characterized by progressive non-hereditary development of multiple bilateral renal cysts in patients on chronic dialysis. It has been reported in 10–20% of patients on dialysis for up to 3 years, 40–60% at 5 years, and in 80–90% of patients who have been on dialysis for 10 years. The cystic development is seen in both peritoneal dialysis and hemodialysis and is independent of the underlying cause of renal failure.[39]

These cysts can cause local hemorrhage, infection, and the development of RCC, which has been reported in 3–7% of patients with ACDK.

Grossly, the involved kidney contains multiple cysts ranging between 0.5 and 3.0 cm in diameter (Figure 3.13) that can be seen usually in the cortex but also in the medulla as dialysis continues. Renal tumor (papillary RCC in more than 70% of cases) may be seen in some cases.

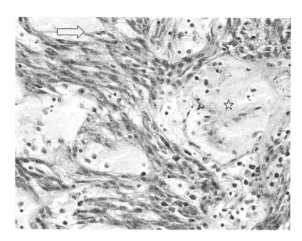

Figure 3.12 Mucinous, tubular, and spindle cell carcinoma showing small tubular formations (arrow), spindle cells, and a pale mucinous stroma (star).

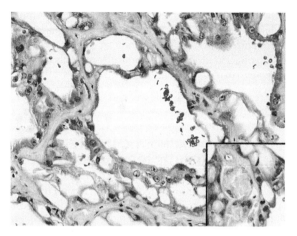

Figure 3.14 Renal cell carcinoma associated with acquired cystic renal disease. This tumor is composed of microcytic space lined by vacuolated, eosinophilic cells. Oxalate crystals can frequently be seen in the cytoplasm of the tumor cells (inset).

MOLECULAR CLASSIFICATION OF RENAL TUMORS

Histopathologic classification (WHO classification), mentioned previously, is critical for clinical management. However, recognition of novel renal tumor subtypes, development of procedures yielding small diagnostic biopsies, and emergence of molecular therapies directed at tumor gene activity make this system more complex. Therefore, gene expression-based classification systems are likely to become essential elements for diagnosis, prognosis, and treatment of patients with RCC.[40]

For RCC, significant achievements in the basic sciences have led to a greater knowledge of the underlying molecular genetics of this disease, which holds the promise of increased sophistication in attempts to tailor patient prognostication and for future treatment strategies. The enhanced ability to predict patient survival will allow for better selection of patients most likely to benefit from systemic therapies and for more accurate comparison of clinical trials based on varying inclusion criteria.

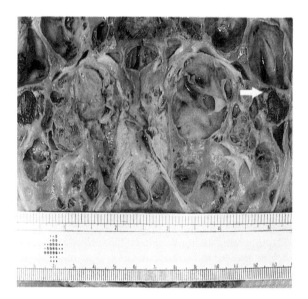

Figure 3.13 Gross appearance of acquired cystic renal disease. Multiple thin-walled cysts are present; the more solid nodule (arrow) turned out to represent a small renal cell carcinoma.

Microscopically, the cysts are lined by flat, cuboidal, hyperplastic, or dysplastic epithelium (Figure 3.14). Renal neoplasm, if present, can be bilateral in 10% of cases and multicentric in 50%. Metastasis has been observed in 20% of such cases.

Currently high-density expression microarrays are expected to provide new molecular diagnostic assays with greater clinical utility for renal tumor classification. These microarrays are solid matrices containing several thousand nucleic acid hybridization targets, representing a large fraction of the entire expressed genome, at fixed addresses. Arrays are probed with labeled cDNA or cRNA, derived from sample mRNA, and then scanned robotically for signal (usually fluorescence) at each hybridization target to quantify the expression of individual genes. Two major microarray platforms are in use: spotted microarrays, containing purified cDNAs or oligonucleotides printed robotically onto glass slides, and microarrays, with short oligonucleotides synthesized directly onto solid substrates using photolithographic or ink-jet techniques.[41–43]

MOLECULAR DIAGNOSTIC MARKERS AND THEIR THERAPEUTIC IMPLICATIONS

The potential of microarray technology in clinical research is enormous. This technology can be used for cancer diagnosis; identification of diagnostic markers through screening and comparing gene and/or protein expression profiles from normal, premalignant, and malignant tissues from the same organ; and the identification of gene and/or protein sets associated with metastasis or response to treatment. Gene and/or protein expression profiles can be derived through microarray technology to allow potentially for diagnosis of a particular cancer and/or of cancer subsets, without examining the histology. This may improve the diagnostic accuracy of current approaches by using immunohistochemical analyses combined with classic histopathologic techniques. Moreover, it is now possible to predict clinical outcome on the basis of gene and/or protein expression patterns.[44,45] Classification of patients into high-risk and low-risk subgroups on the basis of a prognosis profile may be a useful means of guiding adjuvant therapy in patients. This approach should improve the selection of patients who would benefit from adjuvant systemic treatment, reducing the rate of both overtreatment and undertreatment. It may even be possible to predict which patients will benefit from extirpative surgical procedures. Finally, gene and/or protein expression signatures may be used to predict the clinical response to both conventional and targeted therapies. Current efforts at UCLA are to integrate molecular information from tissue microarrays into the UISS to generate a molecular integrated staging system.[46]

RCC microarray assays have led to the discovery of many novel immunohistochemical markers for each major tumor subtype. Table 3.5 summarizes the renal tumor immunomarkers identified with microarrays.

Many overexpressed genes in RCC tumor tissue have therapeutic implications. Clear cell RCC overexpresses immune response genes, which may be important for the relative responsiveness of clear cell RCC to immunotherapy.[47] In large microarray studies of multiple cancers, it appears that RCC may be distinguished from other tumor types by overexpression of angiogenesis genes and coregulation of vascular endothelial growth factor

and carbonic anhydrase (CA) IX.[48] Microarray studies also have established that stem cell factor receptor (KIT) is overexpressed in chromophobe RCC,[49,50] leading several experts to suggest the use of tyrosine kinase inhibitors for advanced carcinomas of this subtype.

Expression profiles of CAIX, CAXII, gelsolin, phosphatase and tensin homolog deleted on chromosome 10 (PTEN), epithelial cell adhesion molecule (EpCAM), CD10, p53, sodium-potassium adenosine triphosphatase subunits, vimentin, Ki-67, CXC chemokine receptor-4, VEGF ligands, VEGF receptors, androgen receptors, bcl-2, α-catenin, cadherin-6, CA-125 protein, epithelial membrane antigen, CD44, insulin like growth factor-1, caveolin-1, and cyclin A have been examined in RCC.[6] However, at this point these markers must still be considered investigational in nature.[46] In RCC, p53 mutations have been associated with cellular proliferation and decrease in apoptosis. Gelsolin functions to sever actin during cell motility. CAIX and CAXII overexpression is a direct consequence of a VHL mutation, which is found in more than 75% of sporadic clear cell RCCs. PTEN regulates cellular migration, proliferation, and apoptosis. EpCAM is expressed on the cell surface of most carcinomas. In RCC, vimentin staining has previously been identified as an independent predictor of poor prognosis. Increased staining for Ki-67, p53, vimentin, and gelsolin correlated with worse survival, whereas the inverse was true for CAIX, PTEN, CAXII, and EpCAM.

PROGNOSTIC NOMOGRAMS FOR RCC

Several prognostic models have been developed to predict disease recurrence and survival after nephrectomy for non-metastatic RCC, using different covariates, tools (nomograms or prognostic categories), and endpoints.

Nomograms are graphic charts that provide outcome probabilities for individual patients and are mainly used to inform patients of the risks and benefits of a treatment or diagnostic procedure.[51] Their use is increasingly common in oncology, especially urologic oncology, for example, for counseling patients with kidney, prostate, or bladder cancer.

Currently, five prognostic nomograms are available for non-metastatic RCC. A postoperative nomogram proposed by Kattan and colleagues, based on the analysis of a Memorial Sloan-Kettering database, is the most widely used model to predict treatment failure and tumor recurrence after surgery for kidney cancer.[51,52] This nomogram is used to calculate the probability that a patient will be free from recurrence at 5 years of follow-up. The four variables included in the nomogram

Table 3.5 Renal tumor immunomarkers identified with microarrays		
Marker	Function	Localization
Clear cell RCC		
Vimentin	Cytoskeleton	Cytoplasm
Adipophilin	Cell differentiation	Cytoplasm
CD10 antigen	Neutral endopeptidase	Membrane
Glutathione S-transferase alpha	Cell detoxification	Cytoplasm
Papillary RCC		
Alpha methylacyl co-enzyme A racemase	Peroxisomal enzyme	Cytoplasm
Cytokeratin 7	Cytoskeleton	Cytoplasm
Chromophobe RCC and oncocytoma		
Beta defensin-1	Antimicrobial/antitumor agent	Cytoplasm
Parvalbumin	Calcium-binding protein	Cytoplasm
Stem cell factor receptor	Cell differentiation	Membrane
Carbonic anhydrase II	Zinc metalloenzyme	Cytoplasm
Cytokeratin 7	Cytoskeleton	Cytoplasm

RCC, renal cell carcinoma.

are clinical symptoms, histology, tumor size, and 1997 TNM stage. It was applied recently in a six-center European study and found to be more accurate than three other models (the University of California–Los Angeles Integrated Staging System [UISS], Mayo Clinic stage, size, grade, and necrosis [SSIGN] score, and the Yaycioglu model).[53] However, in a recent study the Kattan nomogram showed poor performance in predicting overall RCC recurrence.[54] Other models including the UISS model[7] (mentioned previously) includes the TNM classification, Eastern Cooperative Oncology Group (ECOG) performance status (PS) score, and Fuhrman grade, separately for metastatic and non-metastatic RCC. In this study,[54] patients were categorized into three groups with low, intermediate, and high risk. The endpoint was overall survival. The SSIGN score developed by Frank et al[55] includes tumor stage, tumor size, grading, and necrosis. The endpoint of the SSIGN model is cancer-specific survival. All the previous models assigned postoperative scores. Conversely, Yaycioglu et al[56] and Cindolo et al[57] developed pure preoperative scores taking into account only clinical presentation and clinical size of the renal masses and using disease recurrence-free survival as the endpoint. Only two risk groups were derived. All of these models confirmed their ability to discriminate among categories with a different prognosis, although with a difference in discrimination ability among them.[53]

Until now only clinical and pathologic variables have been retained in modern prognostic equations. Postoperative models appear to be the best indicators of survival. Nevertheless, more powerful and accurate systems need to be developed and validated. It is expected that the combination of the usual prognostic variables (such as stage, grade, performance status (PS), histology, tumor size) with new molecular targets will be the next step in the search for a better integrated prognostic system.

Lam et al[46] performed a multivariate analysis for all RCC molecular markers and included metastatic status (Met) as a covariate and an interaction term for CAIX. Only Met, gelsolin, p53, and Met*CAIX remained significant predictors of survival and were used to create a prognostic model (marker model). Using a similar approach, a prognostic model was constructed using a combination of clinical variables and marker data (clinical/marker model). In a multivariate analysis, CAIX, vimentin, and p53 were statistically significant predictors of survival independent of the clinical variables, T stage, metastatic status, Eastern Cooperative Oncology Group-Performance Status (ECOG-PS), and grade. Both nomograms were calibrated, using bootstrap bias corrected estimates, to be accurate to within 10% of the actual 2-year and 4-year survival rates. The predictive ability of each of the various models was quantified by calculating the concordance index (C-index), which demonstrated that prognostic systems based on protein expression profiles for clear cell RCC perform better than standard clinical predictors. The predictive accuracy of the marker model for RCC was comparable to the UISS, and the clinical/marker model was significantly more accurate than the UISS.

Finally, a clinical/marker model for metastatic clear cell RCC patients was constructed.[58] On univariate Cox regression analysis, CAIX, p53, gelsolin, Ki-67, and CAIX were statistically significant predictors of survival. On multivariate Cox regression analysis, only CAIX, PTEN, vimentin, p53, T category, and PS were retained as independent predictors of disease-specific survival and were used to construct a combined molecular and clinical prognostic model. Although these nomograms are useful for visualizing our predictive models, they need to be validated on independent patient populations before being applied to patient care.[46]

REFERENCES

1. Oberling C, River M, Hagueneau F. Ultrastructure of the clear cells in renal cell carcinomas and its importance for the demonstration of their renal cell origin. Nature 1960; 186: 402–3.
2. Jemal A, Murray T, Ward E et al. Cancer statistics, 2005. CA Cancer J Clin 2005; 55(1): 10–30.
3. Jemal A, Siegel R, Ward E et al. Cancer statistics, 2006. CA Cancer J Clin 2007; 57(1): 43–66.
4. Chow WH, Gridley G, Fraumeni JF Jr et al. Obesity, hypertension, and the risk of kidney cancer in men. N Engl J Med 2000; 343(18): 1305–11.
5. Greene FL, Page DL, Fleming ID et al. AJCC Cancer Staging Manual. New York: Springer-Verlag, 2002: 323–5.
6. Lam JS, Shvarts O, Leppert JT et al. Renal cell carcinoma 2005: new frontiers in staging, prognostication, and targeted molecular therapy. J Urol 2005; 173(6): 1853–62.
7. Zisman A, Pantuck AJ, Dorey F et al. Improved prognostication of renal cell carcinoma using an integrated staging system. J Clin Oncol 2001; 19(6): 1649–57.
8. Zisman A, Pantuck AJ, Figlin RA et al. Validation of the UCLA integrated staging system for patients with renal cell carcinoma. J Clin Oncol 2001; 19(17): 3792–3.
9. Slaton JW, Zisman A, Belldegrun A et al. Validation of UCLA integrated staging system (UISS) as a predictor for survival in patients undergoing nephrectomy for renal cell carcinoma. J Urol 2002; 167: 192.
10. Han KR, Bleumer I, Pantuck AJ et al. Validation of an integrated staging system toward improved prognostication of patients with localized renal cell carcinoma in an international population. J Urol 2003; 170(6 Pt1): 2221–4.
11. Patard JJ, Kim HL, Lam JS et al. Use of the University of California Los Angeles integrated staging system to predict survival in renal cell carcinoma: an international multicenter study. J Clin Oncol 2004; 22(16): 3316–22.
12. Zisman A, Pantuck AJ, Wieder J et al. Risk group assessment and clinical outcome algorithm to predict the natural history of patients with surgically resected renal cell carcinoma. J Clin Oncol 2002; 20(23): 4559–66.
13. Lam JS, Belldegrun AS, Figlin RA. Tissue array-based predictions of pathobiology, prognosis, and response to treatment for renal cell carcinoma therapy. Clin Cancer Res 2004; 10(18 Pt2): 6304–9S.
14. Eble JN, Sauter G, Epstein JI et al. World Health Organization Classification of Tumors. Pathology and Genetics of Tumours of the Urinary System and Male Genital Organs. Lyon: IARC Press, 2004.
15. Lopez-Beltran A, Scarpelli M, Montironi R et al. 2004 WHO classification of the renal tumors of the adults. Eur Urol 2006; 49(5): 798–805.
16. MacLennan GT, Resnick MI, Bostwick DG. Pathology for Urologists. Philadelphia: WB Saunders Co, 2003: 1–32.
17. Diaz JI, Mora LB, Hakam A. The Mainz Classification of Renal Cell Tumors. Cancer Control 1999; 6(6): 571–9.
18. Fuhrman SA, Lasky LC, Limas C. Prognostic significance of morphologic parameters in renal cell carcinoma. Am J Surg Pathol 1982; 6(7): 655–63.
19. Cheville JC, Lohse CM, Zincke H et al. Comparisons of outcome and prognostic features among histologic subtypes of renal cell carcinoma. Am J Surg Pathol 2003; 27(5): 612–24.
20. Kovacs G, Fuzesi L, Emanuel A et al. Cytogenetics of papillary renal cell tumors. Genes Chromosomes Cancer 1991; 3(4): 249–55.
21. Schmidt L, Duh FM, Chen F et al. Germline and somatic mutations in the tyrosine kinase domain of the MET protooncogene in papillary renal carcinomas. Nat Genet 1997; 16(1): 68–73.
22. Delahunt B, Eble JN. Papillary renal cell carcinoma: a clinicopathologic and immunohistochemical study of 105 tumors. Mod Pathol 1997; 10(6): 537–44.
23. Gunawan B, von Heydebreck A, Fritsch T et al. Cytogenetic and morphologic typing of 58 papillary renal cell carcinomas: evidence for a cytogenetic evolution of type 2 from type 1 tumors. Cancer Res 2003; 63(19): 6200–5.
24. Thoenes W, Storkel S, Rumpelt HJ. Human chromophobe cell renal carcinoma. Virchows Arch B Cell Pathol Incl Mol Pathol 1985; 48(3): 207–17.
25. Crotty TB, Farrow GM, Lieber MM. Chromophobe cell renal carcinoma: clinicopathological features of 50 cases. J Urol 1995; 154(3): 964–7.
26. Speicher MR, Schoell B, du Manoir S et al. Specific loss of chromosomes 1, 2, 6, 10, 13, 17, and 21 in chromophobe renal cell carcinomas revealed by comparative genomic hybridization. Am J Pathol 1994; 145(2): 356–64.
27. Cohen HT, McGovern FJ. Renal cell carcinoma. N Engl J Med 2005; 353(23): 2477–90.
28. Thoenes W, Sterkel S, Rumpelt HJ et al. Chromophobe cell renal carcinoma and its variants: a report on 32 cases. J Pathol 1988; 155(4): 277–87.
29. Peyromaure M, Misrai V, Thiounn N et al. Chromophobe renal cell carcinoma: analysis of 61 cases. Cancer 2004; 100(7): 1406–10.
30. Rumpelt HJ, Sterkel S, Moll R. Bellini duct carcinoma: further evidence for this rare variant of renal cell carcinoma. Histopathology 1991; 18(2): 115–22.
31. Fuzesi L, Cober M, Mittermayer C. Collecting duct carcinoma: cytogenetic characterization. Histopathology 1992; 21(2): 155–60.
32. Srigley JR, Eble JN. Collecting duct carcinoma of kidney. Semin Diagn Pathol 1998; 15(1): 54–67.
33. Chao D, Zisman A, Pantuck AJ et al. Collecting duct renal cell carcinoma: clinical study of a rare tumor. J Urol 2002; 167(1): 71–4.
34. Davis CJ Jr, Mostofi FK, Sesterhenn IA. Renal medullary carcinoma: the seventh sickle cell nephropathy. Am J Surg Pathol 1995; 19(1): 1–11.

35. Argani P, Lal P, Hutchinson B et al. Aberrant nuclear immuno-reactivity for TFE3 in neoplasms with TFE3 gene fusions: a sensitive and specific immunohistochemical assay. Am J Surg Pathol 2003; 27(6): 750–61.

36. Koyle MA, Hatch DA, Furness III PD et al. Long-term urological complications in survivors younger than 15 months of advanced stage abdominal neuroblastoma. J Urol 2001; 166(4): 1455–8.

37. Rakozy C, Schmahl GE, Bogner S et al. Low-grade tubular-mucinous renal neoplasms: morphologic, immunohistochemical, and genetic features. Mod Pathol 2002; 15(11): 1162–71.

38. Zisman A, Chao DH, Pantuck AJ et al. Unclassified renal cell carcinoma: clinical features and prognostic impact of a new histological subtype. J Urol 2002; 168(3): 950–5.

39. Tickoo SK, dePeralta-Venturina MN, Harik LR et al. Spectrum of epithelial neoplasms in end-stage renal disease: an experience from 66 tumor-bearing kidneys with emphasis on histologic patterns distinct from those in sporadic adult renal neoplasia. Am J Surg Pathol 2006; 30(2): 141–53.

40. Young AN, Dale J, Yin-Goen Q et al. Current trends in molecular classification of adult renal tumors. Urology 2006; 67(5): 873–80.

41. Hughes TR, Mao M, Jones AR et al. Expression profiling using microarrays fabricated by an ink-jet oligonucleotide synthesizer. Nat Biotechnol 2001; 19(4): 342–7.

42. Schena M, Shalon D, Davis RW et al. Quantitative monitoring of gene expression patterns with a complementary DNA microarray. Science 1995; 270(5235): 467–70.

43. Lockhart DJ, Dong H, Byrne MC et al. Expression monitoring by hybridization to high-density oligonucleotide arrays. Nat Biotechnol 1996; 14(13): 1675–80.

44. Kim HL, Seligson D, Liu X et al. Molecular prognostic modeling using protein expression profile in clear cell renal carcinoma. J Urol 2004; 171: 436.

45. Takahashi M, Rhodes DR, Furge KA et al. Gene expression profiling of clear cell renal cell carcinoma gene identification and prognostic classification. Proc Natl Acad Sci USA 2001; 98(17): 9754–9.

46. Lam JS, Leppert JT, Figlin RA et al. Role of molecular markers in the diagnosis and therapy of renal cell carcinoma. Urology 2005; 66(5 Suppl): 1–9.

47. Motzer RJ, Bacik J, Mariani T et al. Treatment outcome and survival associated with metastatic renal cell carcinoma of non-clear-cell histology. J Clin Oncol 2002; 20(9): 2376–81.

48. Amatschek S, Koenig U, Auer H et al. Tissue-wide expression profiling using cDNA subtraction and microarrays to identify tumor-specific genes. Cancer Res 2004; 64(3): 844–56.

49. Higgins JP, Shinghal R, Gill H et al. Gene expression patterns in renal cell carcinoma assessed by complementary DNA microarray. Am J Pathol 2003; 162(3): 925–32.

50. Furge KA, Lucas KA, Takahashi M et al. Robust classification of renal cell carcinoma based on gene expression data and predicted cytogenetic profiles. Cancer Res 2004; 64(12): 4117–21.

51. Hixson ED, Kattan MW. Nomograms are more meaningful than severity-adjusted institutional comparisons for reporting outcomes. Eur Urol 2006; 49(4): 600–3.

52. Kattan MW, Reuter V, Motzer RJ et al. A postoperative prognostic nomogram for renal cell carcinoma. J Urol 2001; 166(1): 63–7.

53. Cindolo L, Patard JJ, Chiodini P et al. Comparison of predictive accuracy of four prognostic models for nonmetastatic renal cell carcinoma after nephrectomy: a multicenter European study. Cancer 2005; 104(7): 1362–71.

54. Hupertan V, Roupret M, Poisson JF et al. Low predictive accuracy of the Kattan postoperative nomogram for renal cell carcinoma recurrence in a population of French patients. Cancer 2006; 107(11): 2604–8.

55. Frank I, Blute ML, Cheville JC et al. An outcome prediction model for patients with clear cell renal cell carcinoma treated with radical nephrectomy based on tumour stage, size, grade and necrosis: the SSIGN score. J Urol 2002; 168(6): 2395–400.

56. Yaycioglu O, Roberts WW, Chan T et al. Prognostic assessment of nonmetastatic renal cell carcinoma: a clinically based model. Urology 2001; 58(2): 141–5.

57. Cindolo L, de La Taille A, Messina G et al. Preoperative clinical prognostic model for non-metastatic renal cell carcinoma. BJU Int 2003; 92(9): 901–5.

58. Kim HL, Seligson D, Liu X et al. Using tumor markers to predict the survival of patients with metastatic renal cell carcinoma. J Urol 2005; 173(5): 1496–501.

4

Imaging renal masses: current status

Vincent G Bird

INTRODUCTION

Renal masses exist in a variety of both solid and cystic forms. They may be detected as a result of specific patient complaints or physical findings, or as part of an evaluation for laboratory findings such as hematuria. With increasing frequency, imaging investigations, initiated due to non-specific or constitutional complaints, are revealing small 'incidental' renal masses of indeterminate biologic nature. These incidental masses pose new challenges to urologists and have introduced the consideration of a larger array of treatment regimens that includes a variety of minimally invasive options.

Renal masses are readily detected by a variety of imaging modalities; however, it is the specific characterization of these masses that is of critical importance. Imaging findings greatly impact clinical decision-making, in terms of whether surgical intervention is necessary, and if so, whether a radical or nephron-sparing approach will be used, and whether an open or minimally invasive approach will be used. Another aim of imaging for renal masses is for the purpose of preoperative staging, as malignancy is likely in the majority of these newly discovered renal lesions. Important aspects of staging that are considered at time of imaging of a renal mass include local extent of tumor, adequate assessment of tumor size, presence of lymph nodes, presence of any tumor-associated thrombus within the renal vein and vena cava, and presence or evidence of possible visceral metastases.

Table 4.1 includes an overview of the differential diagnosis of the most common and some less common renal masses. As is true with most organ structures, a large variety of rare tumors are found in association with the kidney, for which exhaustive lists can be found elsewhere.

RENAL CYSTS

The most common of all renal masses are simple renal cysts, which are characterized by the presence of a thin smooth wall, without irregularity, and having fluid within them. Renal cysts comprise greater than 70% of all asymptomatic renal masses. Solitary or multiple renal cysts are found in more than 50% of patients older than 50 years. Simple renal cysts can be reliably diagnosed by ultrasonography (US), computerized tomography (CT), and magnetic resonance imaging (MRI) and only require treatment rarely, should they become symptomatic.[1,2]

COMPLEX RENAL CYSTS

Aside from simple renal cysts, there is a variety of complex cystic masses, which present their own dilemma, as their probability of harboring malignancy is somewhat difficult to predict. Some cases of complex renal cysts involve some of the most difficult treatment decisions that urologists must make together with their patients. As such, this matter merits significant attention.

Classification schemes, based on specific image-related findings, have been devised in order to help both physicians and patients understand the relative probability that any given cystic mass may harbor malignant renal tumor. Bosniak first introduced his classification of renal cysts in 1986, and has since made refinements in its use.[3] The Bosniak renal cyst classification was first developed based on CT findings. However, it has been applied to other imaging modalities, namely US and MRI. Bosniak does not recommend that ultrasonography be relied upon for differentiation of surgical from non-surgical complex cystic renal masses. However, he feels that MRI is useful for characterizing complex cystic renal masses because lesion vascularity, manifesting as enhancement,

Table 4.1 Renal masses
Renal cyst
Simple
Complex (Bosniak II, III, and IV)
Adenoma
Oncocytoma
Angiomyolipoma
Nephroblastoma (Wilm's tumor)
Transitional cell carcinoma
Renal cell carcinoma
Clear cell
Papillary
Granular
Chromophobe
Collecting duct
Sarcomatoid
Renal medullary
Metastases
Other
Sarcomas
Hemangiopericytoma
Leiomyoma

can be evaluated. Furthermore, it has been shown that the Bosniak classification can be applied to MRI in a reliable manner.[4]

The Bosniak classification system is in widespread use by both urologists and radiologists and is clinically quite practical. The currently used classification scheme is shown in Table 4.2.[5] Using the lesion's morphology and enhancement characteristics, each cystic renal lesion can be categorized into one of five groups (categories I, II, IIF, III, and IV), each with associated recommendations for patient treatment.[5–8] Recent modifications include the use of the IIF category. Follow-up study has shown that many lesions that are well marginated, contain multiple hairline thin septa, have minimal smooth thickening of their wall or septa without measurable enhancement, or contain calcifications, which can be thick, nodular, and irregular, are often benign and as such can be followed.[9] Upon follow-up imaging, any further changes in findings for the lesion in question may then merit surgical intervention. Follow-up study has also shown that the presence of thick, nodular, and irregular calcification is not as significant as once thought. Rather, it is the presence of associated enhancement which appears to increase the risk of malignancy in such lesions.[9,10] The most important parameter in the Bosniak

classification system is the presence of enhancement. The most important criterion used to differentiate surgical lesions from non-surgical lesions is the presence or absence of tissue vascularity, which generally manifests on imaging as enhancement. The association of this finding with malignant cystic lesions is the chief reason why many feel that US alone is not adequate in the evaluation of such lesions. Category III and IV lesions are mainly characterized by enhancement.

The goal of the Bosniak classification scheme is to identify those cystic masses with a reasonably high probability of being malignant and thus minimizing the number of benign renal masses that are removed. Category II lesions are generally benign, and can be followed with periodic renal imaging. Statistical probability for malignancy is approximately 50% for category III lesions. Category IV lesions are mostly all malignant tumors.[11]

Biopsy of a renal mass is often entertained as another means to differentiate surgical from non-surgical cystic lesions, however there are a number of studies that point to the lack of reliability or need for doing so in the majority of cases.[12–16] Furthermore, although reportedly rare, biopsy of a neoplastic lesion can cause needle tumor seeding and, in cystic masses, potential spillage and implantation of malignant cells.[14,17]

ENHANCING RENAL MASSES

Solid enhancing renal masses are obviously of great concern in that there is reasonably high probability of their harboring malignancy. However, renal masses with mostly solid elements tend to have a constellation of radiologic findings that do not reliably correlate with the histopathologic features of these masses, which as aforementioned more often than not are malignant. It is for this reason that solid renal masses are considered malignant until proven otherwise.

Most clinical decisions regarding renal masses are largely based on the findings of imaging. As such, it is of primary importance to understand what types of imaging modalities are available and how reliable each modality is in terms of detection of renal masses and further ascertaining the potential for malignancy based upon modality-specific measurable parameters. Though it may appear apparent the more advanced imaging modalities such as CT and MR are often superior in terms of the characterization of renal masses, it is important to understand in the larger clinical context that applications of these modalities have their own inherent limitations in terms of cost, availability, and contraindications. Contrast toxicity due to allergy or pre-existing renal insufficiency may preclude CT with intravenous contrast administration.

Category	Description
Table 4.2 Bosniak classification for cystic renal masses[5]	
I	A benign simple cyst with a hairline thin wall that does not contain septa, calcifications, or solid components. It measures water density and does not enhance
II	A benign cyst that may contain a few hairline thin septa in which `perceived´ enhancement may be present. Fine calcification or a short segment of slightly thickened calcification may be present in the wall or septa. Uniformly high attenuation lesions <3 cm (so-called high-density cysts) that are well marginated and do not enhance are included in this group. Cysts in this category do not require further evaluation
IIF (F for follow-up)	Cysts that may contain multiple hairline thin septa or minimal smooth thickening of their wall or septa. Perceived enhancement of their septa or wall may be present. Their wall or septa may contain calcification that may be thick and nodular, but no measurable contrast enhancement is present. These lesions are generally well marginated. Totally intrarenal non-enhancing high-attenuation renal lesions >3 cm are also included in this category. These lesions require follow-up studies to prove benignity
III	'Indeterminate' cystic masses that have thickened irregular or smooth walls or septa in which measurable enhancement is present. These are surgical lesions, although some will prove to be benign (e.g., hemorrhagic cysts, chronic infected cysts, and multiloculated cystic nephroma), some will be malignant, such as cystic renal cell carcinoma and multiloculated cystic renal cell carcinoma
IV	These are clearly malignant cystic masses that can have all the criteria of category III, but also contain enhancing soft-tissue components adjacent to, but independent of, the wall or septum. These lesions include cystic carcinomas and require surgical removal

Existence of certain implanted metallic devices may preclude MRI. In only a minority of cases do specific findings of imaging and factors related to specific patient history give impetus to the performance of renal mass biopsy in order to further guide clinical decision-making.

IMAGING MODALITIES

Anatomic imaging modalities historically used for the characterization of renal masses include intravenous contrast-enhanced plain film radiography, US, CT, and MRI. Intravenous contrast-enhanced plain film radiography and CT both expose patients to ionizing radiation, which is within acceptable risk parameters, and involve the use of intravenous iodinated contrast agents, which carry an albeit low, but real risk. Iodinated contrast media entail risk in three types of ways: (1) a metabolic effect relating to their hypertonicity, (2) inducement of acute renal dysfunction, and (3) idiosyncratic contrast material reactions. These issues are addressed here.

Plain film radiography and CT require the use of ionizing radiation. Advances in radiation technology and

equipment design have resulted in lower dose and overall exposure, but total exposure is additive. Total exposure to ionizing radiation for every patient should be considered, as there are carcinogenic risks associated with exposure to large cumulative doses of radiation. Total exposure to radiation is measured in a number of different ways. Dose may be measured as both skin dose and total effective radiation dose. Effective absorbed radiation, in sieverts, can also be measured. Analysis of a number of studies suggests that a three-phase CT scan exposes patients to approximately two to three times as much radiation as approximately 12 plain film radiographs (which may be more than are used at many institutions for many patients) taken during the course of intravenous pyelography.[18–20] As more advanced CT protocols use more runs, this issue is of concern. Recommendations for limiting radiation in these studies include eliminating a phase (which may then limit examination accuracy) or reducing mA during some of the phases of the study.[21]

Risks associated with hypertonicity include increased cardiac output and decreased peripheral vascular resistance due to volume expansion,[22] inhibition of the coagulation cascade by high osmolar contrast agents,[23] and renovascular dilation followed by renovascular constriction, with a resulting decrease in glomerular filtration rate.[24]

Acute impairment in renal function (increase in serum creatinine of 0.5 to 1.0 mg/dl or 25–50% decrease in the glomerular filtration rate) occurs in 1/1000–5000 patients without known risk factors. This condition is generally non-oliguric; however, when it is accompanied by oliguria, a risk of permanent renal damage exists.[25,26] Risk factors that increase the risk of acute renal dysfunction include pre-existing renal insufficiency, diabetic nephropathy, congestive heart failure, hyperuricemia, proteinuria, and multiple administrations of contrast material in a short time period.[27] General recommendations to avoid acute renal dysfunction include ample pre-examination hydration, avoidance of dehydrating preparations, and a reduction in total contrast used, if feasible.

Patients who take metformin for control of diabetes mellitus are advised to stop this medication 48 hours prior to contrast administration. When renal function and urine output are demonstrated to be normal after imaging, metformin therapy may be resumed. The concern for these patients is that if acute renal dysfunction occurs during metformin administration, they may develop significant lactic acidosis.[28]

Idiosyncratic contrast material reaction, the third type of contrast-related risk, may occur in mild, moderate, and severe forms. Mild reactions include metallic taste, sensation of warmth, sneezing, coughing, and mild urticaria. Moderate reactions include vomiting, more severe urticaria, headache, edema, and palpitations. These reactions can be symptomatically treated as needed. However, severe reactions, which include hypotension, bronchospasm, laryngeal edema, pulmonary edema, and loss of consciousness, require immediate intervention.[29] Fortunately, severe reactions occur in less than 0.1% of patients, and it is estimated that 80% of these may be avoided by the use of low osmolar contrast media.[30,31]

All contrast-associated risks appear to be lowered by the use of low osmolar contrast media that are now available. Administration of prophylactic corticosteroids and use of low osmolar contrast media have been shown to decrease the risk of contrast reaction, but not eliminate it.[32] Methylprednisolone 32 mg oral may be given every 12 hours starting 24 hours prior to examination. This may be continued for 12–24 hours after the examination to ensure that all contrast material has been excreted.[33] Diphenhydramine 50 mg orally may also be administered before contrast administration. All patients offered intravenous iodinated contrast studies should be counseled and informed of these associated risks.

Contrast-enhanced plain film radiography

The IVP, or intravenous pyelogram (also IVU – intravenous urogram), has long been a mainstay of the urologist's diagnostic armamentarium. This test requires the use of intravenous iodinated contrast. This test generally requires bowel preparation for optimal imaging results, an absence of patient contraindications to intravenous iodinated contrast administration, repeated imaging over 30 to 60 minutes, and at times more prolonged imaging if renal obstruction is present.

After a scout film is taken, contrast is injected, at which time nephrotomograms are obtained. These images may reveal abnormalities of the renal parenchyma. However, recent studies comparing IVP to other imaging modalities, namely CT, show that sensitivity for detection and characterization of renal masses is limited. Findings suggestive of a mass seen on IVP generally require other types of imaging for both corroboration and specific delineation.

When performed properly, intravenous pyelography provides valuable information pertaining to the pyelocalyceal system, including the existence of hydronephrosis, hydroureteronephrosis, existence of urinary stones, and 'filling defects', which include a variety of diagnostic possibilities. However, there is concern that IVP has limited sensitivity for renal parenchymal pathologies. Previous studies have documented the limited sensitivity of small renal masses, particularly when masses are less than 3 cm.[34–37] CT urography has gained great popularity in that it provides reliable assessment of both the renal parenchyma and collecting system. In a prospective comparison of CT and excretory urography in the initial evaluation of microscopic hematuria, Sears et al demonstrated that initial examination with CT had a better diagnostic yield for a wide variety of pathologies.[34]

In summary, IVP has fallen out of favor at many institutions for a variety of reasons that include risk of contrast toxicity, time consumption involved in performance of the test, and limited diagnostic accuracy in triage setting where diagnoses are often still uncertain.

Ultrasonography

Ultrasound as an imaging option is immediately attractive as the exam requires neither contrast administration nor ionizing radiation. Its mechanism of action is based on the transmission of a pulse of high frequency sound energy into the patient. These sound waves are then either reflected, refracted, or absorbed, depending on what type of tissue is encountered. The ultrasound transducer also acts as a receiver, which receives the returning echoes. The collected input is processed by a computer for the creation of a composite image.[29] Ultrasound is now performed in a real-time manner which allows for the technician and physician to modify and review different aspects of the examination. Newer machines also have significantly improved resolution.

Ultrasonography is used widely throughout many medical specialties. It may be used by anyone with proper training and experience in almost any clinical scenario: radiology suite, clinic, and under sterile conditions in the operating room. The applications of US are so extensive that they cannot be enumerated here (Figure 4.1). However, with this said, it should be made clear to those evaluating any imaging performed with this modality that this is an operator-dependent test. As such, if the individual charged with interpretation of the images is not present during the actual real-time study, and is undecided as to interpretation of the still images, the study may need to be repeated if that itself is feasible. Image quality is also closely related to the quality of equipment being used.

Ultrasonography of a large number of different body structures is performed with the use of a variety of probes depending on parameters that include patient body habitus and structures to be imaged. In the case of the kidney, 3.5 to 5 MHz transducers are typically used. Transducers of this range are used to obtain adequate depth of penetration without substantial loss of resolution. Bony structures and bowel gas may both interfere with renal imaging, more so on the left than the right.

Ultrasound is commonly employed as an initial imaging exam due to its relatively low cost of performance, ease of performance, and lack of significant risk associated with its performance. The strength of US is its ability to differentiate solid versus cystic renal structures. In the hands of an experienced ultrasonographer, it is quite reliable for the identification and confirmation of simple renal cysts; however, as is the case with IVP, there is concern regarding low sensitivity for detection of small renal masses.[35,37] However, there are proponents who claim that well-performed duplex US may be quite accurate in the diagnosis and staging of a large number of renal masses, including those cases where renal vein or caval thrombus are involved. There are limitations in respect to the identification of lymphadenopathy, which also is a limitation in cases where CT is employed.[38] In addition to its many other uses, US of the kidney remains a very useful imaging modality and still has a large role in renal imaging in patients with azotemia, those with severe contrast allergy, pregnant patients, neonates, and children. Ultrasonography may at times be quite useful for assessment of renal masses in the intraoperative setting, both for open cases and laparoscopic cases. In the open setting it may be useful for the identification of relatively small masses completely hidden within the renal parenchyma, or in cases where multiple small tumors, not all of which are immediately amenable to manual palpation, are suspected. Laparoscopic ultrasound may be useful in a similar fashion, and may also be used in concert with different ablative devices that are at times used in the treatment of select renal masses.

In terms of differentiation of solid renal masses using US, the presence of shadowing, a hypoechoic rim, and intratumoral cysts are thought to be important findings that may help distinguish angiomyolipomas from other solid lesions, namely renal cell carcinoma.[39] Nonetheless, these findings are not reliable enough to make such a diagnosis with reasonable certainty.

More recently, contrast-enhanced US has been introduced as another means of further characterizing renal masses. Ultrasound contrast agents are injected as liquids, and then undergo a phase change to a gas when in the bloodstream. This contrast agent, in its gas form, improves the detection of Doppler signals and helps better reveal both normal and abnormal vascularity.[40] In this type of ultrasound study, the contrast agent is injected, and when evident on imaging, the patient holds their breath while a number of ultrasound frames are obtained for analysis. Proponents put forth that contrast-enhanced US entails less risk than contrast-enhanced CT and can show even subtle tumor blood flow, and may serve as a viable alternative for patients unable to undergo contrast enhanced CT or MRI for any variety of reasons.[41] To date there appears to be only limited use of this augmented form of US. More experience with it is necessary in order to assess what future role it may serve.

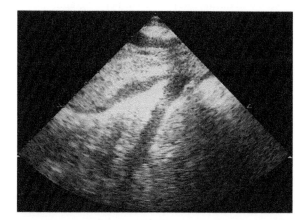

Figure 4.1 Ultrasound is very versatile. This view is taken from a transesophageal probe. It demonstrates a large inferior vena cava thrombus traversing the diaphragm and entering the right atrium (courtesy of Gaetano Ciancio MD).

Computerized tomography

The advent of CT was a significant event in the evolution of abdominal imaging. Similar to plain film radiography, images obtained by this modality are created due to the attenuation of photons by the body tissue being examined. A thin collimated X-ray beam is generated on one side of the patient. Detectors on the opposite side of the patient then measure the amount of transmitted radiation. In any given transverse plane being examined these measurements are repeated as the X-ray beam rotates around the patient. During processing, the measurements are taken and placed into a matrix of CT values that correspond to the attenuation of a given tissue volume within the patient. The gray scale of each CT pixel is related to the amount of radiation absorbed at that point. This value is called the attenuation value, and is commonly denoted in Hounsfield units. Clinically relevant CT Hounsfield unit values are shown in Table 4.3.[29]

These obtained measurements are then taken from a given transverse slice of body tissue and are mathematically processed by a computer that then reconstructs a cross-sectional image of the body. Conventional CT scanners obtain transverse images one slice at a time. However, more recently evolved spiral (or helical) CT scanners allow movement of the patient on a gantry with simultaneous tunnel rotation with continuous X-ray exposure. This arrangement allows for rapid acquisition of volumetric data from the patient being examined during the time in which breathing is being suspended. The acquisition of volumetric data is of great value in terms of renal imaging in that it allows for greater accuracy and detail in terms of evaluating renal parenchymal masses and renal vasculature, particularly in terms of visualization of small renal masses and supernumerary renal blood vessels. Data acquired in this manner also allow for high quality CT angiography and three-dimensional reconstructions in a variety of ways[29] (Figure 4.2).

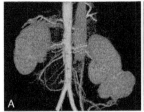 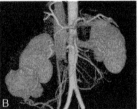

Figure 4.2 Acquisition of volumetric data now allows for CT reconstructions such as this three-dimensional spatial model of the kidneys, associated tumors, and vasculature. (A) Anterior view; (B) posterior view.

Contrast-enhanced CT provides excellent anatomic detail for retroperitoneal structures and as such has become the mainstay for radiologic diagnosis of renal masses. Distinct phases have been clearly identified for patients undergoing intravenous contrast-enhanced renal imaging. These phases include the arterial, corticomedullary, nephrographic, and excretory ones. The arterial phase occurs approximately 15–25 seconds after contrast administration. It is most useful for the identification of renal arterial anatomy and is generally most useful for evaluating renal donors and those with suspected renovascular pathologies. The corticomedullary phase occurs approximately 25–70 seconds after injection. During this phase the renal cortex has intense enhancement, as glomerular filtration of the contrast material begins to take place. This phase is useful for the identification of hypervascular renal tumors, notably clear cell renal cell carcinomas. The renal veins can also be seen well during this phase. The nephrographic phase generally occurs 80–120 seconds after contrast administration. During this phase contrast has been filtered through the glomeruli and has made its way to the collecting ducts. The renal parenchyma appears homogeneous during this phase. It is at this time that subtle renal parenchymal masses are best detected. The last phase, the excretory phase, generally occurs 180 seconds after contrast administration. During this phase the renal calyces, pelvis, and ureters are opacified. At times, further delayed imaging is necessary to ensure that all portions of the ureter have been opacified.[42]

Most recently, advanced protocols for contrast-enhanced CT have been employed with the intention of gathering as many data as possible for a given renal mass. These protocols are directed toward differentiation of hyperdense cysts, complex cysts, and various types of solid renal masses, i.e. oncocytomas, angiomyolipomas, and subtypes of renal cell carcinoma. These protocols often entail the identification of a region of interest within the mass in question, and then recording its density,

Table 4.3 Hounsfield values[29]	
Absorber	**CT numbers (HUs)**
Bone	+1000
Calculus	+400 or greater
Calcification	+160 or greater
Acute hemorrhage	+50 to 90
Soft tissue	+10 to 50
Water	0
Fat	−100
Air	−1000

in Hounsfield units, throughout the various phases of the study, which include the non-contrast phase and the aforementioned contrast-enhanced phases.

Though not exclusively specific, certain types of renal masses tend to have relatively common features on contrast-enhanced CT. Angiomyolipomas often have fat components, which appear as low attenuation regions (generally negative Hounsfield units). However, fat-poor angiomyolipomas may not show such features. Milner et al noted that cases involving less than 25% fat/high-power field on histologic analysis correlated with CT findings where fat usually was not noted.[43] Oftentimes, oncocytomas may show a low attenuation 'central scar' within the mass in question. This finding, however, is not particularly useful in that many oncocytomas are not associated with this finding, and at times may co-exist with renal cell carcinoma as well.

Histologic subtypes of renal cell carcinoma may often have characteristic enhancement 'signatures' on multi-phase contrast-enhanced CT. Clear cell renal cell carci-nomas are often quite vascularized, and often have high Hounsfield unit values in the early phases of the study immediately following contrast administration. Papillary renal cell carcinomas are relatively hypovascular and generally show mild enhancement during the study. Peak enhancement for papillary renal cell carcinomas may continue to increase during the latter corticomedullary and delayed phases of the study (Figures 4.3 and 4.4).

CT scanners are undergoing a continuing evolution. Newer generation scanners have larger numbers of detectors that exist in a variety of configurations. These multidetector configurations allow for images of differ-ent slice thickness during image acquisition. Additional detectors also allow for more helices to be generated. The most recently produced scanners have 32 rows of detectors, which allow for rapid imaging and more precise imaging of smaller masses. Scanners with even more rows of detectors are already being produced. This evolution may continue with even newer paradigms of detection that include an image plate detector. It is believed that this new advance may further improve imaging of very small structures, such as small renal masses and small renal blood vessels. Such technology may also result in less volume averaging and pixilation, factors that often limit imaging of small renal masses.[44]

Magnetic resonance imaging

Magnetic resonance imaging is the most recent of anatomic imaging modalities instituted for renal imaging. The mechanism of MRI requires extensive description, but essentially involves placement of the patient within a magnetic field, which results in the alignment of the hydrogen protons in their body tissue. This alignment

leads to the formation of a magnetic vector. This vector can be made to spin with the application of radiofre-quency pulse. A wire (coil) outside the patient will then have a current induced within it by the magnetic force. At this point the current emanating from the body tissue can be measured. The magnitude of this current is related to the intensity of the pixel in the MR image.[45] MR information can be processed for the creation of direct multiplanar images, i.e., transverse, sagittal, and coronal (the latter two not possible with CT). Due to its nature, MR may yield particularly unique information regarding blood flow and fluid composition, which is useful in a variety of circumstances, namely the identi-fication of fluid and blood in renal cysts and tumor-associated renal vein/inferior vena cava thrombus (Figure 4.5). Contraindications to performance of MRI include those with pacemakers, ferromagnetic intracra-nial aneurysm clips, cochlear implants, metallic ocular foreign bodies, and some particular makes of older pros-thetic heart valves. Early MR scanners had practical imaging problems in that breath holding was often nec-essary for proper data acquisition. New generation scan-ners, with more rapid acquisition times, have allowed for much more practical and reasonable patient breath holding, thus adding to the practicality of regular use of this modality.

In relation to contrast-enhanced MRI, it is important to understand that gadolinium, a paramagnetic lan-thanide metal, the agent used in conjunction with chelates as an MR contrast agent, is quite different from the iodine-based contrast material used in plain film radi-ography and CT. It is not nephrotoxic.[46] Gadolinium-based MR contrast agents are associated with less allergic reactions than iodinated contrast agents.[47] Gadolinium-based contrast agents are safe for use both in patients with limited renal function and those with a history of allergic reaction to iodinated contrast material.[48–50] This makes MRI very attractive for use in the assessment of renal disorders in children, women of childbearing age, patients with renal insufficiency, and those with renal allografts.[51]

Contrast of different body tissue on MR examination is quite different from that of CT. Important factors include proton density, T1 and T2 and magnetic sus-ceptibility, and flow. In brief, T1 is a measure of how quickly a tissue can become magnetized and T2 relates to how quickly a given body tissue loses its magnetiza-tion. MR protocols for renal masses vary slightly, but essentially include precontrast T1 and T2 fast spin echo sequences, where elements of assessment include dis-cerning the presence of fat (bright T1 signal), hemor-rhage (bright T1 signal), and cystic lesions (bright T2 signal).[29] Axial acquisition is preferred as comparison to CT images is often done. A similar technique should

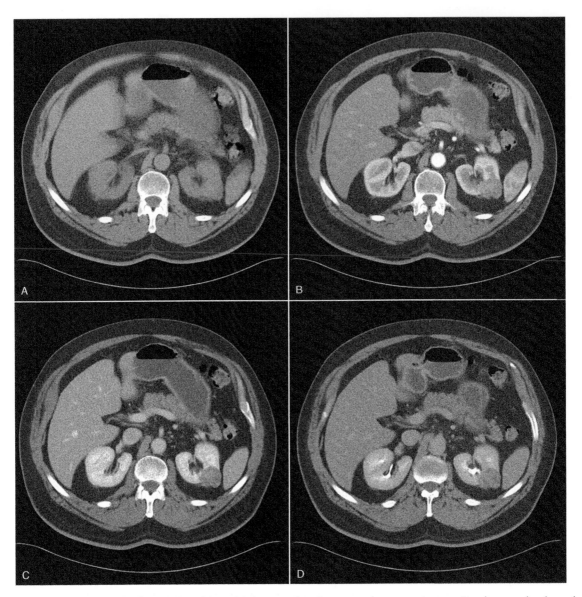

Figure 4.3 (A)–(D) Multiphase CT. In this multiphase study a hypovascular tumor is seen. It enhances slowly and less so than the surrounding normal renal parenchyma, a pattern noted to be consistent with papillary renal cell carcinoma. Pathologic analysis revealed this tumor to be a papillary renal cell carcinoma.

be used during the precontrast and contrast-enhanced portions of the exam to allow for proper comparison. Other techniques, such as frequency-selective fat-suppression techniques (FATSAT) or chemical shift (in- and out-of-phase) help distinguish the presence of fat from that of hemorrhage in a renal lesion. Specific techniques are also used to assess for flow defects within the renal vein and inferior vena cava. Images acquired in the axial plane generally yield the best vascular images as well. A cardiac synchronized sequence can be used if initial techniques are inconclusive in cases of determination of the presence of renal vein/inferior vena cava thrombus (thrombus results in a persistent filling defect over the entire cardiac cycle).[52]

On MRI, enhancement is measured in terms of signal intensity. Similar to CT, motion artifact, volume

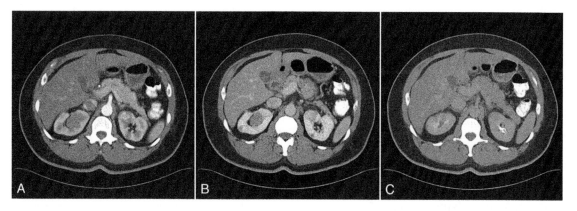

Figures 4.4 (A)–(C) Subtle tumors may not be optimally visualized during the corticomedullary phase. However, this tumor is readily seen during the nephrographic phase. Pathologic analysis revealed this tumor to be a clear cell renal cell carcinoma.

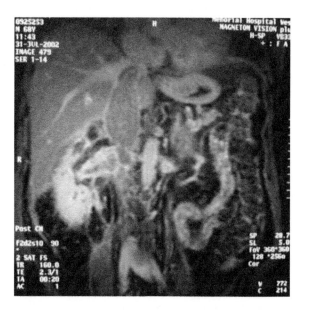

Figure 4.5 MR coronal view of extensive renal vein and inferior cava thrombus (courtesy of Gaetano Ciancio MD).

averaging, and fluctuations in signal intensity may result in pseudoenhancement. For a 0.1 mmol/kg contrast dose on a 1.5 T MR scanner 15% enhancement over the baseline precontrast signal has been considered 'significant' enhancement, though it is important to understand that this value may not be applicable to other scanners, field strengths, and imaging techniques.[52]

MRI is useful for differentiation of solid renal masses and cysts, much like its less expensive counterparts, CT and US. Due to reasons related to cost and availability,

urologic evaluations with MRI are generally reserved for patients with iodinated contrast toxicity, limited renal function, masses still regarded as indeterminate on CT scan, and cases where there is adequate suspicion for renal vein/inferior vena cava thrombus. MRI is considered excellent for vascular structures and the liver, and as such is considered both necessary and useful in cases where the possible presence of renal vein and inferior vena cava tumor-associated thrombus needs to be assessed. Various MR techniques may be used to assess for fat within renal tumors, however, as is the case with CT, fat-poor angiomyolipomas exist and thus make specific radiologic diagnosis of this entity less than certain.

As has been done with CT scanning, attempts have been made to use differential intensity of signal enhancement with MRI in order to aid differentiation of benign versus malignant masses, namely differentiating benign oncocytomas from malignant renal cell carcinomas. However, protocols used to date have not been able to reliably differentiate these two groups of tumors.[53]

COMPARING COMPUTERIZED TOMOGRAPHY AND MAGNETIC RESONANCE IMAGING

Comparison of CT and MR is rather complex in that they are actually two distinct imaging modalities. Though, certainly, each one has its distinct merits and advantages.

CT and MR scanners have both evolved in terms of provision of improved or more advanced images. Overall, both are equally successful in terms of detection and staging of renal masses.[54,55] In a review comparing CT and MRI of cystic renal masses, Israel et al noted that though both modalities were of equal value in the majority of cases, in certain instances MR depicted additional septa, presence of wall thickening, or enhancement that resulted in upgrading of the Bosniak cyst classification, which may then impact management decisions. However, pathologic correlation was not available for all lesions.[56] Thus, at this time, it remains unclear whether one modality is more useful than the other in this respect.

However, it does appear that MRI is better for evaluation of venous invasion by tumor thrombus.[52,54,56] MR is quite useful for the assessment of tumor involvement of vascular structures and overall tumor extent, due to its unique ability to assess vascular flow and its being readily amenable to repeated image acquisition in a variety of tissue planes. MRI also does not require the use of ionizing radiation, a difference that becomes considerably more obvious when advanced MR and CT techniques, which require multiple passes, are compared. MR also has clear benefits in those patients who are at risk of morbidity from intravenous iodinated contrast administration for one of a variety of reasons.[52]

On the other hand, ease of use, speed, overall anatomic coverage, and image preference all favor CT. Practicality and time consumption for imaging are large economic factors and are a continuing impetus for many institutions to obtain newer ever faster CT scanners. Moreover, advanced reconstruction programs used with these new CT scanners that can rapidly acquire large volumes of volumetric data now allow for more advanced imaging previously considered not possible with this modality.

Many advantages may be perceived or be readily appreciated by the urologist, radiologist, or the institution that owns and operates these scanners, but not necessarily by all of them. Urologists generally have a longer and greater experience with CT, and are familiar with CT images. However, urologists may be relatively less familiar with the large variety of advanced MR techniques that radiologists can use that helps characterize renal lesions. Even so, studies to date performed by both radiologists and urologists, using both of these modalities, have not resolved the dilemma of being able to reliably differentiate benign and malignant enhancing masses. Healthcare institutions and providers consider a variety of factors relating to issues of economics and availability of resources. It remains to be seen whether the application of new protocols to either modality, or the advent of new technologies or enhancements to these devices, will shed any further light on preference of use of these two imaging modalities.

Interest in differentiation of solid and benign renal masses by means of imaging has continued. A recent study suggests that smaller masses do have a relatively higher chance of being benign, or if malignant, are of relatively low grade.[57] This same study suggests that larger, higher-stage symptomatic masses are more likely to be malignant than those that are asymptomatic. However, this type of statistical information is still only of limited value in the clinical consideration of a given renal mass in a given patient. Perhaps the consideration of new imaging paradigms, such as that of positron emission tomographic scanning, using tumor-specific binding agents, can be used in conjunction with anatomic imaging, and will one day allow for both anatomic and biologic description of renal masses.

REFERENCES

1. Novick AN, Campbell SC. Renal tumors. In: Walsh PC, Retik AB, Vaughan ED Jr, Wein AJ, eds. Campbell's Urology 8th Edition, Philadelphia: Saunders, 2002: 2672–731.
2. Kissane JN. The morphology of renal cystic disease. In: Gardner KD, ed. Cystic Diseases of the Kidney. New York: Wiley and Sons, 1976: 31.
3. Bosniak MA. The current radiological approach to renal cysts. Radiology 1986; 158: 1–10.
4. Israel GM, Hindman N, Bosniak MA: Comparison of CT and MRI in the evaluation of cystic renal masses. Radiology 2004; 231: 365–71.
5. Israel GM, Bosniak MA. An update of the Bosniak renal cyst classification system. Urology 2005; 66(3): 484–8.
6. Curry NS, Cochran ST, Bissada NK. Cystic renal masses accurate Bosniak classification requires adequate renal CT. AJR Am J Roentgenol 2000; 175: 339–42.
7. Koga S, Nishikido M, Inuzuka S et al. An evaluation of Bosniak's radiological classification of cystic renal masses. BJU Int 2000; 86: 607–9.
8. Levy P, Helenon O, Merran S et al. Cystic tumors of the kidney in adults radio-histopathologic correlations. J Radiol 1999; 80: 121–33.
9. Israel GM, Bosniak MA. Follow-up CT studies for moderately complex cystic renal masses (Bosniak category IIF). Am J Roentgenol 2003; 181: 627–33.
10. Israel GM, Bosniak MA. Calcification in cystic renal masses: is it important in diagnosis? Radiology 2003; 226: 47–52.
11. Siegel CL, Middleton WD, Teefey SA et al: Angiomyolipoma and renal cell carcinoma: US differentiation. Radiology 1996; 198(3): 789–93.
12. Renshaw AA, Granter SR, Cibas ES. Fine-needle aspiration of the adult kidney. Cancer 1997; 81: 71–88.
13. Dechet CB, Zincke H, Sebo TJ et al. Prospective analysis of computerized tomography and needle biopsy with permanent sectioning to determine the nature of solid renal masses in adults. J Urol 2003; 169: 71–4.
14. Bosniak MA. Should we biopsy complex cystic renal masses (Bosniak category III)? Am J Roentgenol 2003; 181: 1425–6.
15. Hayakawa M, Hatano T, Tsuji A et al. Patients with renal cysts associated with renal cell carcinoma and the clinical implications of cyst puncture: a study of 223 cases. Urology 1996; 47: 643–6.
16. Horwitz CA, Manivel JC, Inampudi S et al. Diagnostic difficulties in the interpretation of needle aspiration material from large renal cysts. Diagn Cytopathol 1994; 11: 380–3.
17. Herts BR, Baker ME. The current role of percutaneous biopsy in the evaluation of renal masses. Semin Urol Oncol 1995; 13: 254–61.
18. Herts BR. The current status of CT urography. Crit Rev Comput Tomogr 2002; 43: 219–41.

19. McTavish JD, Jinzaki M, Zou KH et al. Multi-detector row CT urography: comparison of strategies for depicting the normal urinary collecting system. Radiology 2002; 225: 783–90.

20. Caoili EM, Cohan RH, Korobkin M et al. Urinary tract abnormalities: initial experience with multi-detector row CT urography. Radiolgy 2002; 222: 353–60.

21. Noroozian M, Cohan RH, Caoili EM et al. Multislice CT urography: state of the art. Br J Radiol 2004; 77: S74–86.

22. Morris TW. The physiologic effects of nonionic contrast media on the heart. Invest Radiol 1993; 28: S44–6.

23. Stormorken H, Skalpe IO, Testart MC. Effects of various contrast media on coagulation, fibrinolysis, and platelet function: an in vitro and in vivo study. Invest Radiol 1986; 21: 348–54.

24. Porter GA. Effects of contrast agents on renal function. Invest Radiol 1993; 28: S1–5.

25. Porter GA. Contrast media-associated nephrotoxicity. Recognition and management. Invest Radiol 1993; 28: S11–8.

26. Mudge GH. Nephrotoxicity of urographic radiocontrast drugs. Kidney Int 1980; 18: 540–52.

27. Barrett BJ, Carlisle EJ. Meta-analysis of the relative nephrotoxicity of high and low osmolality iodinated contrast media. Radiology 1993; 188: 171.

28. Thompsen HS, Morcos SK. Contrast media and metformin: guideline to diminish the risk of lactic acidosis in noninsulin dependent diabetics after administration of contrast agents. Eur Radiol 1999; 9: 738–40.

29. Schulam PG, Kawashima A, Sandler C et al. Urinary tract imaging – basic principles. In: Walsh PC, Retik AB, Vaughan Jr ED, Wein AJ eds. Campbell's Urology 8th Edition, Philadelphia: Saunders, 2002: 122–66.

30. Katayama H, Yamaguchi K, Kozuka T et al. Adverse reactions to ionic and nonionic contrast media. Radiology 1990; 175: 621–8.

31. Caro JJ, Trindade E, McGregor M. The risks of death and of severe nonfatal reactions with high vs low-osmolality contrast media: a meta-analysis. Am J Roentgenol 1991; 156: 825–32.

32. Greenberger PA, Patterson R. The prevention of immediate generalized reactions to radiocontrast media in high-risk patients. J Allergy Clin Immunol 1991; 87: 867–72.

33. Lasser EC, Berry CC, Mishkin MM et al. Pretreatment with corticosteroids to prevent adverse reactions to nonionic contrast media. Am J Roentgenol 1994; 162: 523–6.

34. Sears CL, Ward JF, Sears ST et al. Prospective comparison of computerized tomography and excretory urography in the initial evaluation of asymptomatic microhematuria. J Urol 2002; 168: 2457–60.

35. Warshauer DM, McCarthy SM, Street SM et al. Detection of renal masses: sensitivities and specificities of excretory urography/linear tomography, US, and CT. Radiology 1988; 169: 363.

36. Dikranian AH, Pettiti DB, Shapiro CE et al. Intravenous urography in evaluation of asymptomatic microhematuria. J Endourol 2005; 19(5): 595–7.

37. Lang E, Macchia RJ, Thomas R et al. Improved detection of renal pathologic features on multiphasic helical CT compared with IVU in patients presenting with microscopic hematuria. Urology 2003 61(3): 528–32.

38. Bos SD, Mensink HJ. Can duplex Doppler ultrasound replace computerized tomography in staging patients with renal cell carcinoma? Scand J Urol Nephrol 1998; 2: 87–91.

39. Israel GM, Bosniak MA. Renal imaging for diagnosis and staging of renal cell carcinoma. In: Taneja SS, ed. Contemporary management of Renal Cell Carcinoma. Philadelphia: WB Saunders Co., 2003, 30: 499–514.

40. Girard MS, Mattrey RF, Baker KG et al. Comparison of standard and second harmonic B-mode sonography in the detection of segmental renal infarction with sonographic contrast in a rabbit model. J Ultrasound Med 2000; 19: 185–92.

41. Tamai, H, Takiguchi Y, Oka M et al. Contrast-enhanced ultrasonography in the diagnosis of solid renal tumors. J Ultrasound Med 2005; 24: 1635–40.

42. Sheth S, Fishman EK. CT in Kidney Cancer. Imaging of Kidney Cancer. New York: Springer Berlin Heidelberg 2006: 29–49.

43. Milner J, McNeil B, Alioto J et al. Fat poor renal angiomyolipoma: patient, computerized tomography and histological findings. J Urol 176(3): 905–9.

44. Lockhart ME, Smith K. Technical considerations in renal CT. In: Kenney PJ, ed. Radiologic Clinics of North America – Advances in Renal Imaging. Philadelphia, Pennsylvania, W. B. Saunders Company, 2003; 41(5): 863–75.

45. Dunnick NR, Sandler CM, Amis Jr ES, Newhouse JH. Textbook of Uroradiology. Baltimore, Maryland. Williams & Wilkins, 1997: 44–85.

46. Terens WL, Gluck R, Golimbu M et al. Use of gadolinium DTPA-enhanced MRI to characterize renal mass in patient with renal insufficiency. Urology 1992; 40: 152–4.

47. Nelson KL, Gifford LM, Lauber-Huber C et al. Clinical safety of gadopentate dimeglumine. Radiology 1995; 196: 439–43.

48. Nelson KL, Gifford LM, Lauber-Huber C et al. Clinical safety of adopentatedimeglumine. Radiology 1995; 196: 439–3.

49. Prince MR, Arnoldus C, Frisoli JK: Nephrotoxicity of high dose gadolinium compared with iodinated contrast. J Magn Reson Imaging 1996; 6: 162–6.

50. Rofsky NM, Weinreb JC, Bosniak MA et al. Renal lesion characterization with gadolinium-enhanced MR imaging: efficacy and safety in patients with renal insufficiency. Radiology 1991; 180: 85–9.

51. Zhang J, Pedrosa I, Rofsky NM: MR techniques for renal imaging. In Kenney PJ. ed. Radiologic Clinics of North America – Advances in Renal Imaging. Philadelphia, Pennsylvania, W. B. Saunders Company, 2003; 41(5): 877–907.

52. Ho VB, Choyke PL. MR evaluation of solid renal masses. In Lee VS ed. Magnetic Resonace Imaging Clinics of North America – Genitourinary MR Imaging. Philadelphia. W. B. Saunders. 2004; 12: 413–27.

53. Hecht EM, Israel GM, Krinsky GA et al. Renal masses: quantitative analysis of enhancement with signal intensity measurements versus qualitative analysis of enhancement with image subtraction for diagnosing malignancy at MR imaging. Radiology 2004; 232: 373–8.

54. Hallscheidt P, Stolte E, Roeren T et al. The staging of renal-cell carcinomas in MRI and CT – a prospective histologically controlled study. Rofo Fortschr Geb Rontgenstr Neuen Bildgeb Verfahr 1998; 168(2): 165–70.

55. Walter C, Kruessell M, Gindele E et al. Imaging of renal lesions: evaluation of fast MRI and helical CT. Br J Radiol 2003; 76(910): 696–703.

56. Israel GM, Hindman N, Bosniak MA: Evaluation of cystic renal masses: Comparison of CT and MR imaging by using the Bosniak classification system. Radiology 2004; 231: 365–71.

57. Schlomer B, Figenshau R, Yan Y et al. Pathological features of renal neoplasms classified by size and symptomatology. J Urol 2006; 176: 1317–20; discussion 1320.

5

Hypothermia and renoprotective measures in nephron-sparing surgery

Ming-Kuen Lai

INTRODUCTION

Renal cell carcinoma (RCC) is the most common cancer of newly diagnosed malignancies in the kidney. Elective nephron-sparing surgery (NSS), i.e., partial nephrectomy for patients with a small (generally defined as less than 4 cm in diameter), localized RCC is associated with a low risk of local recurrence (0–3%) and excellent cancer-specific survival rates (90–100%).[1,2] Nowadays, many cases of benign and malignant renal tumors are detected at early stage through the wide use of non-invasive imaging techniques such as ultrasonography. NSS is becoming more important than ever.

In either open partial nephrectomy (OPN) or laparoscopic partial nephrectomy (LPN),[3,4] a certain period of renal ischemia via occlusion of the renal artery and then reperfusion of the renal parenchyma after the occlusion is released is involved in the majority of cases. Ischemia/reperfusion injury (IRI) to the renal parenchyma is one of the major concerns in NSS. In humans, 30 minutes is the maximum tolerable period of warm ischemia before permanent damage takes place. Although temporary arterial occlusion during NSS is generally believed not to affect short-term renal function adversely,[5,6] a reduction in the renal function of the operated kidney by a mean of 29% has been reported.[7] Old age and pre-existing azotemia increase the risk of renal damage after LPN, especially when the warm ischemia exceeds 30 minutes. Hypothermia and renoprotective measures are urgently needed in such cases.

Hypothermia is commonly used to protect the kidneys from IRI. Lowering the renal temperature reduces energy-dependent metabolic activity and slows down oxygen and ATP consumption. Hypothermia with a uniform kidney temperature of 20–25°C is adequate to maintain renal function even after 3 hours of arterial occlusion.[8] Renal cooling through an angiographic catheter in the renal artery,[9] a ureteral catheter in the pelvicalyceal system,[10,11] with a coil,[12] or by using ice slush in a laparoscopic bag[13] for LPN have been reported. No reliable and effective method is yet available for laparoscopic renal cooling that can match the level of renal cooling achieved with ice slush in open partial nephrectomy.

RENAL ISCHEMIA AND REPERFUSION INJURY

Ischemia/reperfusion injury is a series of complicated reactions which involve the vascular endothelium and activated leukocytes.[14] Dysfunction of these structures leads to vascular congestion, diminished blood flow, and leukocyte infiltration. Mononuclear cell infiltration and the presence of peritubular T lymphocytes have been identified in experimental IRI. The signal transduction in apoptotic cell death and the contribution of various molecular components of these pathways in IRI have been studied extensively.[15] Global gene expression has been studied in IRI using oligonucleotide microarrays. Genes involved in extracellular matrix–cell interactions and cell–cell interactions were found to be upregulated.[16] During the early phase of reperfusion, P-selectin is rapidly released onto the cell surface. ICAM-1, which is constitutively expressed on the surface of endothelial cells, is involved in neutrophil adhesion.[17] Apoptosis and necrosis often occur simultaneously in IRI. Initiator caspases (e.g., caspase-8 and caspase-9) proteolytically activate effector caspases (e.g., caspase-3 and caspase-7), which express catalytic properties to dissolve the cell and carry out the final steps of the apoptotic cell destruction.[18]

The hypoxic condition leads to deprivation of vital energy elements and loss of ATP storage in the nephron of the outer medullary region. After the ischemic insults, even though the total renal blood flow returns to normal, marked regional derangements occur. There are various degrees of vascular and tubular dysfunction as a result of IRI. The endothelial cells become swollen, leaky, activated, and cannot function normally.[19] Damage occurs predominantly to the most distal segment (S3) of the proximal tubules, leading to proximal tubular cell (PTC) dysfunction. The S3 segments that locate in the outer medulla are extremely susceptible to ischemic injury. This is because of their low glycolytic capacity to regenerate ATP when ATP is depleted rapidly and the oxidative phosphorylation process is impaired. Sodium and potassium pumps, which are supported by ATP, become impaired during ischemia and lead to loss of electrolyte gradients across the cell membrane. Cellular edema occurs after such an event. The better availability of ATP in the distal tubule cells makes them less vulnerable to injury and apoptotic cell death under severe stress conditions.[20] Products of ATP breakdown are normally converted to urea by xanthine dehydrogenase. Under ischemic conditions, xanthine dehydrogenase is converted to xanthine oxidase. This process takes approximately 30 minutes in renal tissue. During the reperfusion phase, in the presence of oxygen, xanthine oxidase will convert the accumulated products into xanthine and the superoxide anion, a free radical which in turn will cause peroxidation and cellular destruction.[21]

Reactive oxygen species (ROS) are oxygen related free radicals which are produced within a few minutes of reperfusion and continuously to be generated for hours after restoration of blood flow to the ischemic tissue. ROS include: superoxide anion ($\bullet O_2$), hydrogen peroxide (H_2O_2), hypochlorous acid (HOCL), nitric oxide-derived peroxynitrite, hydroxyl radical ($\bullet OH$). Prolonged ischemia enhances proapoptotic machinery, including increases in the Bax/Bcl-2 ratio, CPP32 expression, and poly-(ADP-ribose)-polymerase fragments, and subsequently results in apoptosis in renal tubules in a time-dependent fashion. In tubular cell cultures, significant increases in apoptotic cells are evident in PTCs after IRI. The oxidative damage in PTCs, but not in distal tubular (DT) cells, can be alleviated by ROS scavengers, e.g., superoxide dismutase (SOD) and hexa(sulfobutyl)fullerene, a powerful free radical scavenger. These findings confirm that PTCs are vulnerable to ROS.[22] IRI in the kidney is associated with the generation of ROS in the neutrophils and in parenchymal cells, e.g., proximal tubules and endothelial cells. ROS are chemically reactive and ready to oxidize membrane lipids, proteins, and nucleic acids, and eventually will lead to loss of cell function. There are various sources related

to the production of ROS including the mitochondrial electron transport chain, xanthine oxidase, lipoxygenases, and cyclooxygenases.[23] ROS are important in mediating IRI. ROS induce damage to the cells by peroxidation of lipid membranes, protein denaturation, and DNA strand breaks.[24] Extensive DNA damage associated with IRI leads to excessive activation of the DNA repair enzyme PARP[25] and ATP depletion.[26]

Treatment with free radical scavengers, such as SOD, dimethylthiourea, and many experimental free radical scavengers attenuates ischemic acute renal failure.[27–30] Antioxidants or free radical scavengers are used clinically to prevent or decrease renal IRI injury, e.g., in the renal preservative solution.[31] The most commonly used preservative solutions for kidney transplantation are the UW solution[32,33] and Euro-Collins solution. However, they are not applicable to NSS due to their high potassium content, which is dangerous or lethal if it leaks inadvertently into the systemic circulation.

Nitric oxide (NO) is a free radical derived from the oxidation of the guanidino group of L-arginine under the control of NO synthase (NOS). Three isoforms of NOS have been described and cloned: brain NOS (bNOS, nNOS, or type 1), inducible macrophage-type NOS (iNOS or type 2), and endothelial cell NOS (eNOS or type 3). Reperfusion rapidly induces large amounts of NO in the renal proximal tubules through upregulation of iNOS from activated leukocytes, vascular smooth muscle cells, or endothelial cells.[34,35] NO is important in renal homeostasis, e.g., by maintaining renal blood flow and glomerular filtration rate. However, NO has been shown to be involved in the pathogenesis of IRI.[36] Induction of iNOS may have either toxic or protective effects. The superoxide can react with nitric oxide and form peroxynitrite, which is a precursor of the highly toxic hydroxyl free radical.[36,37] Peroxynitrite actively nitrates protein tyrosine residues to form nitrotyrosine adducts, alters protein function, and causes reperfusion injury. A considerable portion of the toxic effects attributed to NO or ROS might be modulated by peroxynitrite. Peroxynitrite instead of NO may be the ultimate cytotoxic substance in IRI.[38]

In some preservative solutions, nitroglycerin as NO donor and L-arginine as substrate for endogenous NO synthase are added in the ingredients.[31] NO augmentation has been shown to be beneficial in several experimental models of heart and lung, renal, and liver transplantation.[39] Various techniques that are being developed include the use of antisense oligonucleotides,[37] recombinant proteins, small molecules to disrupt protein–protein interactions, and caspase inhibitors.[40] Antisense strategies are used to modulate the expression of Bcl-XL, c-FLIP, and survivin.[41] Caspase inhibitors using components mimicking peptide ketones have provided valuable information.[40,42] Specific caspase inhibitors might be valuable in treating various acute injuries such as IRI in NSS.[41] Release of cytochrome C from the mitochondria can be triggered by Bax, which has been shown to trigger cell death. The anti-apoptotic effect of Bcl-2 can block cytochrome C release and caspase activation, and can render ischemic tissue more resistant to reperfusion-induced oxidative stress.[43] My colleagues and I have reported a method of gene delivery with adenovirus vector which transfers bcl-2 genes to the kidneys. The Bcl-2-augmented renal tubules can protect against IRI through the antioxidant and anti-apoptotic actions.[44]

RENAL PRESERVATION IN NEPHRON-SPARING SURGERY

The procedure of renal preservation includes methods of hypothermia, in situ renal preservation with different perfusates, and pharmacologic agents to prevent postischemic renal failure and reperfusion injury (IRI).

Methods of hypothermia

Hypothermia to slow down oxygen consumption and ATP depletion is an effective method of organ preservation. Reduced temperature suppresses metabolism: metabolism is decreased 1.5–2-fold for every 10°C decrease in temperature.[45] In an animal study, the optimum temperature for renal hypothermia was found to be 15°C.[46] Several studies have shown that there is no additional protection from renal cell injury due to ischemia by cooling below 15°C, hence this is recommended as the optimum temperature for use in clinical renal hypothermia.[46] The preservative solution further protects the kidney by preventing unfavorable shifts in electrolytes, solutes, and water into the cell, thereby preventing harmful cell swelling.[47] However, commercially available preservative solutions cannot be used in NSS due to their high potassium content. Renal cooling with a uniform temperature of 20–25°C is adequate to maintain renal function even after 3 hours of arterial occlusion.[8] Newer potassium–titanyl–phosphate laser techniques might offer the performance of partial nephrectomy without pedicle clamping and hypothermia management.[48]

Methods of renal cooling through an angiographic catheter in the renal artery,[9] a ureteral catheter in the pelvicalyceal system,[10,11] with a coil,[12] or by using ice slush in a laparoscopic bag[13] are currently used in NSS. The details, pros, and cons of each method will be discussed in the following sections.

Cooling through an angiographic catheter in the renal artery

In 1978, Marberger et al[49] reported simultaneous intraluminal balloon occlusion of the renal artery and intermittent hypothermic perfusion in open kidney surgery. The double-lumen, balloon-tipped catheter was introduced into the renal artery percutaneously prior to the operation. External surface cooling may lower the kidney temperature heterogeneously while hypothermic perfusion through the renal artery can achieve a more homogeneous hypothermia. Transarterial hypothermic renal perfusion seems to offer better preservation of renal function than topical ice slush hypothermia.[50] The disadvantage of this technique is the necessity of preoperative insertion of the angiographic catheter by a radiologist. The tip of the angiocatheter might slip out of the renal artery during the process of transportation to the operative room or positioning for insertion of the ureteral catheter. The risk of tumor cell spillage is not increased through this technique because the perfusion flow and pressure are less than in the normal circulation.

Masaki et al[51] reported a technique of hypothermic perfusion with cold Euro-Collins solution through a cannula which was inserted into the renal artery through arteriotomy of the segmental artery supplying the renal tumor, while the venous blood and perfusate were drained from the left gonadal vein or a small venotomy incision of the right renal vein. This technique seems to be too complicated for a laparoscopic procedure. Janetschek et al[9] reported a technique to occlude the renal artery with a ballooned angiographic catheter, however it did not achieve an effective occlusion. A tourniquet for an arterial occlusion proved to be much safer. The angiographic catheter was used only for cold perfusion with iced Ringer's lactate at 4°C at a rate of 50 ml per minute.

We use a 5 to 5.5 Fr balloon angiographic catheter positioned in the renal artery for both pedicle control and cold perfusion with chilled Ringer's lactate solution in which vitamin C is added for further renal protection during laparoscopic partial nephrectomy. N-Acetylcysteine 600 mg orally twice daily is given one day before the operation. Between 15 and 30 g of mannitol solution is infused 30 minutes before the renal artery is occluded. Diuresis and hyperosmolarity of the renal parenchyma after mannitol infusion render the kidney less vulnerable to IRI. The mannitol infusion can be repeated after the arterial occlusion is released. More than 10 cases have been performed in such a manner. The technique proved to be safe and effective. In the case illustrated in Figure 5.1, a small tumor was located near the renal hilum (A). Because the image study could not differentiate between angiomyolipoma and renal cell carcinoma, LPN was performed. During the

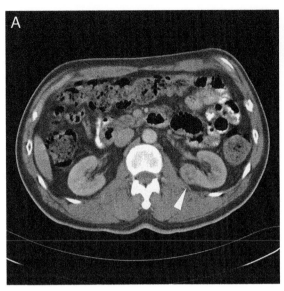
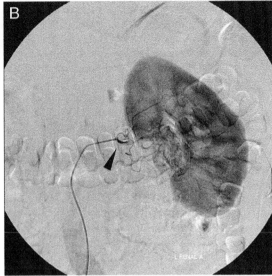

Figure 5.1 A small tumor (white arrowhead) was located near the left renal hilum (A). Angiographic catheter (arrowhead) was introduced into left renal artery (B). During the process of hemostatic suturing, the occlusion balloon was repeatedly released and re-occluded to check for adequate hemostasis and ensure that the renal pedicles were not compromised.

process of hemostatic suturing, the occlusion balloon (B) was repeatedly released and re-occluded to check for adequate hemostasis and to ensure that the renal pedicles were not compromised. The angiographic catheter was left in position overnight in case of further bleeding. It could be re-inflated if necessary. The catheter was removed on the following day, after the risk of further bleeding had subsided.

Cooling through a ureteral catheter in the pelvicalyceal system

Landman et al[10] reported a technique using a ureteral access sheath and a 7.1 Fr pigtail catheter which was advanced inside the sheath. Ice-cold saline ($-1.7°C$) was circulated through the access sheath and drained via the pigtail catheter. A renal cortical temperature of 24°C and a medullary temperature of 21°C could be achieved. In the porcine model study,[11] although renal hypothermia could be achieved by transureteral iced saline infusion, external cooling by using ice slush was more efficient. Intrarenal cooling via a transureteral approach may allow more effective cooling of the renal medulla and decrease warm ischemia during laparoscopic partial nephrectomy. This technique can be combined with cooling through an angiographic catheter in the renal artery, as described above, to further ensure adequate renal cooling.

Cooling with a coil or by using ice slush

Herrell et al[52] described a technique of cooling the kidney with sterile gloves modified into bags that have been filled with sterile ice slush. These gloves are placed around the kidney through the hand assisted device. Porcine model experiments confirmed the efficacy of such an approach in achieving protective hypothermic temperatures (15°C). Gill et al[13] reported a similar technique, which cooled the kidney with an Endocatch (Auto Suture Company, UK) bag filled with ice slush.

The preservative solution

From the early works by Collins et al,[53] it was realized that the kidney has to be rapidly flushed and cooled using a preservative solution to minimize enzymatic activity and energy substrate depletion. The flush solution was formulated to resemble the intracellular fluid, i.e., high potassium and magnesium concentrations, rather than the extracellular ionic content.[53] University of Wisconsin (UW) solution is the standard preservative solution used for abdominal organ transplantation. The histidine–tryptophan–ketoglutarate (HTK) solution, developed in the 1970s by Bretschneider et al as a cardioplegia solution, is being used increasingly for kidney and other organs.[54] UW solution contains metabolically inert substrates, such as lactobinate and raffinose, hydroxyethyl starch as a colloid carrier, and adenosine as an energy substrate. Experience in renal transplantation has proved HTK solution and UW solution to be essentially equivalent as preservative solutions. Both solutions have a clear advantage over the Euro-Collins solution.[55] These preservative solutions were designed for ex vivo perfusion; their high potassium concentration makes them unsafe for in situ perfusion unless the perfusate can be drained out totally from the venous end. Clinically, chilled Ringer's lactate solution mixed with mannitol and vitamin C can be used as a flush solution.

Pharmacologic agents to prevent postischemic renal failure and reperfusion injury

Catalytic antioxidants

Superoxide dismutase, glutathione peroxidase (GPX), and catalase are used to detoxify ROS by their dismutation reactions. The use of SOD and catalase as therapeutic agents to attenuate ROS-induced injury might have a theoretic protective effect, however the effect is not consistent as shown by the animal experiments on the lung IRI model.[56–58] Addition of either an oxygen free radical scavenger such as ceruloplasmin or an iron-chelating agent such as deferoxamine to the perfusate has been reported to improve the effect of kidney preservation in animal models.[59] Allopurinol has been reported to reduce Na^+K^+ ATPase-related lipid peroxidation in ischemic and reperfused kidneys.[60] However, data from human applications are still lacking.

The main limitations of these natural products in the treatment of IRI are their large size, which limits cell permeability, their short circulating half-life, their antigenicity as a foreign protein, and their cost. A low molecular weight SOD has been developed to overcome some of these limitations. In addition, the expression of antioxidant genes, e.g., mRNA for catalase, GPX, and CuZnSOD, during ischemia-reperfusion is not consistent and the uncoordinated loss of antioxidant enzymes may contribute to the heterogeneous renal tissue damage as a result of IRI.[61] The efficacy of using these exogenous antioxidants to treat IRI is debatable and not conclusive.

N-Acetylcysteine (NAC) is a thiol-containing antioxidant which has been shown to have a protective effect on kidneys subjected to ischemia-reperfusion.[62] NAC has been used clinically to prevent contrast-medium-induced renal toxicity.[63] The plasma half-life of NAC after intravenous injection is approximately 6 to 40 minutes. Intravenously administered NAC binds extensively to plasma and tissue proteins, forming disulfides. Thus, very little free NAC is found in the circulation after intravenous injection. Oral administration is recommended despite its low oral availability. The therapeutic benefits of oral NAC are probably not direct, but rather secondary effects, e.g., induction of glutathione synthesis. We give NAC 600 mg orally twice daily before surgery. A higher dose regimen with a loading dose of 140 mg/kg followed by repeated doses of 70 mg/kg has been reported.[64] Allopurinol, an inhibitor of xanthine oxidase, has also been reported to have a protective effect against renal IRI. In the rat model, pretreatment with 50 mg/kg allopurinol, given intraperitoneally 5 hours and 1 hour before renal ischemia, has been shown to be protective.[64]

Other supportive pharmacologic agents

A supportive regimen with hydration, vasodilators such as phenoxybenzamine and diuretics such as furosemide, and mannitol contributes to a decrease in the degree of renal IRI. Since cyclooxygenases (COX) 1 and 2 can be detected in tissue submitted to IRI, COX 1 and COX 2 inhibition with indomethacin or rofecoxib can ameliorate the renal tissue damage triggered by IRI in the mouse model.[65]

CONCLUSION

Until the time comes when surgical technique is greatly advanced and pedicle control is not necessary during nephron-sparing partial nephrectomy, renal preservation measurement using hypothermia and protective pharmacologic agents remains to be an important issue. Currently available methods and pharmacologic agents offer some benefits, however they do not provide user-friendly procedures and satisfactory results. Further studies are urgently needed to fulfill the needs.

REFERENCES

1. Novick AC. Nephron-sparing surgery for renal cell carcinoma. Ann Rev Med 2002; 53: 393–407.
2. Sengupta S, Zincke H. Lessons learned in the surgical management of renal cell carcinoma. Urology 2005; 66(Suppl 5A): 36–42.
3. Weld KJ, Venkatesh R, Huang J et al. Evolution of surgical technique and patient outcomes for laparoscopic partial nephrectomy. Urology 2006; 67: 502–6.
4. Haber GP, Gill IS. Laparoscopic partial nephrectomy: contemporary technique and outcomes. Eur Urol 2006; 49: 660–5.
5. Kane CJ, Mitchell JA, Meng MV et al. Laparoscopic partial nephrectomy with temporary artery occlusion. Description of technique and renal functional outcomes. Urology 2004; 63: 241–6.

6. Shekarriz B, Shah G, Upadhyay J. Impact of temporary hilar clamping during laparoscopic partial nephrectomy on postoperative renal function: a prospective study. J Urol 2004; 172(1): 54–7.

7. Desai MM, Gill IS, Ramani AP et al. The impact of warm ischaemia on renal function after laparoscopic partial nephrectomy. Br J Urol Int 2005; 95: 377–83.

8. Ramani AP, Ryndin I, Lynch AC et al. Current concepts in achieving renal hypothermia during laparoscopic partial nephrectomy. Br J Urol Int 2006; 97: 342–4.

9. Janetschek G, Abdelmaksoud A, Bagheri F et al. Laparoscopic partial nephrectomy in cold ischemia: renal artery perfusion. J Urol 2004; 171(1): 68–71.

10. Landman J, Venkatesh R, Lee D. Renal hypothermia achieved by retrograde endoscopic cold saline perfusion: technique and initial clinical application. Urology 2003; 61: 1023–5.

11. Crain DS, Spencer CR, Favata MA et al. Transureteral saline perfusion to obtain renal hypothermia: potential application in laparoscopic partial nephrectomy. J Soc Laparoendoscop Surg 2004; 8: 217–22.

12. Webster TM, Moeckel GW, Herrell SD. Second prize: simple method for achieving renal parenchymal hypothermia for pure laparoscopic partial nephrectomy. J Endourol 2005; 19: 1075–81.

13. Gill IS, Abreu SC, Desai MM et al. Laparoscopic ice slush renal hypothermia for partial nephrectomy: the initial experience. J Urol 2003; 170: 52–6.

14. Weight SC, Bell PRF, Nicholson ML. Renal ischaemia-reperfusion injury. Br J Surg 1996; 83: 162–70.

15. Padanilam BJ. Cell death induced by acute renal injury: a perspective on the contributions of apoptosis and necrosis. Am J Physiol Renal Physiol 2003; 284: F608–27.

16. Yoshida T, Tang SS, Hsiao LL et al. Global analysis of gene expression in renal ischemia-reperfusion in the mouse. Biochem Biophys Res Commun 2002; 91: 787–94.

17. Zhou T, Sun GZ, Zhang MJ et al. Role of adhesion molecules and dendritic cells in rat hepatic/renal ischemia-reperfusion injury and anti-adhesive intervention with anti-P-selectin lectin-EGF domain monoclonal antibody. World J Gastroenterol 2005; 11: 1005–10.

18. Thornberry NA. Caspases: a decade of death research. Cell Death Different 1999; 6: 1023–7.

19. Molitoris BA, Sandoval R, Sutton TA. Endothelial injury and dysfunction in ischemic acute renal failure. Crit Care Med 2002; 30: S235–40.

20. Bonventre JV. Mechanisms of ischemic acute renal failure. Kidney Int 1993; 43: 1160–78.

21. St Peter SD, Imber CJ, Friend PJ. Liver and kidney preservation by perfusion. Lancet 2002; 359: 604–13.

22. Chien CT, Lee PH, Chen CF et al. De novo demonstration and co-localization of free-radical production and apoptosis formation in rat kidney subjected to ischemia/reperfusion. J Am Soc Nephrol 2001; 12: 973–82.

23. Thadhani R, Pascual M, Bonventre JV. Acute renal failure. N Engl J Med 1996; 334: 1448–60.

24. Devalaraja-Narashimha K, Singaravelu K, Padanilam BJ. Poly(ADP-ribose) polymerase-mediated cell injury in acute renal failure. Pharmacol Res 2005; 52(1): 44–59.

25. Martin DR, Lewington AJ, Hammerman MR et al. Inhibition of poly(ADP-ribose) polymerase attenuates ischemic renal injury in rats. Am J Physiol Regul Integr Comp Physiol 2000; 279: R1834–40.

26. Ha HC, Snyder SH. Poly(ADP-ribose) polymerase is a mediator of necrotic cell death by ATP depletion. Proc Natl Acad Sci USA 1999; 96: 13978–82.

27. Singh D, Chopra K. Effect of trimetazidine on renal ischemia/reperfusion injury in rats. Pharmacol Res 2004; 50: 623–9.

28. Doi K, Suzuki Y, Nakao A et al. Radical scavenger edaravone developed for clinical use ameliorates ischemia/reperfusion injury in rat kidney. Kidney Int 2004; 65: 1714–23.

29. Zahmatkesh M, Kadkhodaee M, Moosavi SM et al. Beneficial effects of MnTBAP, a broad-spectrum reactive species scavenger, in rat renal ischemia/reperfusion injury. Clin Exp Nephrol 2005; 9: 212–18.

30. Chatterjee PK, Cuzzocrea S, Brown PA et al. Tempol, a membrane-permeable radical scavenger, reduces oxidant stress-mediated renal dysfunction and injury in the rat. Kidney Int 2000; 58: 658–73.

31. Guarrera JV, Polyak M, Arrington BO et al. Pulsatile machine perfusion with Vasosol solution improves early graft function after cadaveric renal transplantation. Transplant 2004; 77: 1264–8.

32. Faenza A, Catena F, Nardo B et al. Kidney preservation with University of Wisconsin and Celsior solution: a prospective multi-center randomized study. Transplant 2001; 72: 1274–7.

33. Southard JH, Belzer FO. Organ preservation. Ann Rev Med 1995; 46: 235–47.

34. Weight SC, Furness PN, Nicholson ML. Nitric oxide generation is increased in experimental renal warm ischaemia-reperfusion injury. Br J Surg 1998; 85: 1663.

35. Goligorsky MS, Noiri E. Duality of nitric oxide in acute renal injury. Semin Nephrol 1999; 19: 263–71.

36. Lien YH, Lai LW, Silva AL. Pathogenesis of renal ischemia/reperfusion injury: lessons from knockout mice. Life Sci 2003; 74: 543–52.

37. Peresleni T, Noiri E, Bahou WF et al. Antisense oligodeoxynucleotides to inducible NO synthase rescue epithelial cells from oxidative stress injury. Am J Physiol Renal Fluid Electrolyte Physiol 1996; 270: F971–7.

38. Nicholson DW. From bench to clinic with apoptosis-based therapeutic agents. Nature 2000; 407: 810–16.

39. Garcia-Calvo M, Peterson EP, Leiting B et al. Inhibition of human caspases by peptide-based and macromolecular inhibitors. J Biol Chem 1998; 273: 32608–13.

40. Daemen MA, van't Veer C, Denecker G et al. Inhibition of apoptosis induced by ischemia-reperfusion prevents inflammation. J Clin Invest 1999; 104: 541–9.

41. Zhao H, Yenari MA, Cheng D et al. Bcl-2 overexpression protects against neuron loss within the ischemic margin following experimental stroke and inhibits cytochrome c translocation and caspase-3 activity. J Neurochem 2003; 85: 1026–36.

42. Basile DP, Liapis H, Hammerman MR. Expression of bcl-2 and bax in regenerating rat renal tubules following ischemic injury. Am J Physiol 1997; 272: F640–7.

43. Hassem W, Heaton ND. The role of mitochondria in ischemia/reperfusion injury in organ transplantation. Kidney Int 2004; 66(2): 514–17.

44. Chien CT, Chang TC, Tsai CY et al. Adenovirus-mediated bcl-2 gene transfer inhibits renal ischemia/reperfusion induced tubular oxidative stress and apoptosis. Am J Transpl 2005; 5: 1–10.

45. Clavien PA, Harvey PR, Strasberg SM. Preservation and reperfusion injuries in liver allografts: an overview and synthesis of current studies. Transplant 1992; 53: 957–78.

46. Ward JP. Determination of the optimum temperature for regional renal hypothermia during temporary renal ischaemia. Br J Urol 1975; 47(1): 17–24.

47. Hauet T, Goujon JM, Vandewalle A. To what extent can limiting cold ischaemia/reperfusion injury prevent delayed graft function? Nephrol Dial Transplant 2001; 16(10): 1982–5.

48. Moinzadeh A, Gill IS, Rubenstein M et al. Potassium–titanyl–phosphate laser laparoscopic partial nephrectomy without hilar clamping in the survival calf model. J Urol 2005; 174: 1110–14.

49. Marberger M, Georgi M, Guenther R et al. Simultaneous balloon occlusion of the renal artery and hypothermic perfusion in in situ surgery of the kidney. J Urol 1978; 119: 463–7.

50. Marberger M, Eisenberger F. Regional hypothermia of the kidney: surface or transarterial perfusion cooling? A functional study. J Urol 1980; 124: 179–83.

51. Masaki Z, Ichigi Y, Kuratomi K et al. In situ perfusion by retrograde cannulation of a tumor artery for nephron-sparing surgery. Int J Urol 1995; 2: 161–5.

52. Herrell SD, Baldwin DB, Porter J et al. New technique: hand-assisted laparoscopic partial nephrectomy with hypothermia – animal model and early human application. J Endourol 2002; 16: A20.

53. Collins GM, Peterson T, Wicomb WN et al. Experimental observations on the mode of action of 'intracellular' flush solution. J Surg Res 1984; 36: 1–8.

54. Isemer FE, Ludwig A, Schunck O et al. Kidney procurement with the HTK solution of Bretschneider. Transplant Proc 1988; 20: 885–6.

55. Stubenitsky BM, Booster MH, Nederstigt AP et al. Kidney preservation in the next millennium. Transplant Int 1999; 12: 83–91.

56. Simonson SG, Welty-Wolf KE, Huang YC et al. Aerosolized manganese SOD decreases hyperoxic pulmonary injury in primates. I. Physiology and biochemistry. J Appl Physiol 1997; 83: 550–8.

57. Lardot C, Broeckaert F, Lison D et al. Exogenous catalase may potentiate oxidant-mediated lung injury in the female Sprague-Dawley rat. J Toxicol Environ Health 1996; 47: 509–22.

58. Ouriel K, Smedira NG, Ricotta JJ. Protection of the kidney after temporary ischemia: free radical scavengers. J Vascular Surg 1985; 2: 49–53.

59. Baron P, Gomez-Marin O, Casas C et al. Renal preservation after warm ischemia using oxygen free radical scavengers to prevent reperfusion injury. J Surg Res 1991; 51(1): 60–5.

60. Aricioglu A, Aydin S, Turkozkan N et al. The effect of allopurinol on Na$^+$K$^+$ ATPase related lipid peroxidation in ischemic and reperfused rabbit kidney. Gen Pharmacol 1994; 25: 341–4.

61. Dobashi K, Ghosh B, Orak JK et al. Kidney ischemia-reperfusion: modulation of antioxidant defenses. Mol Cell Biochem 2000; 205: 1–11.

62. Conesa EL, Valero F, Nadal JC et al. N-Acetyl-L-cysteine improves renal medullary hypoperfusion in acute renal failure. Am J Physiol Regul Integr Comp Physiol 2001; 281: R730–7.

63. Fishbane S, Durham H, Marzo K et al. N-Acetylcysteine in the prevention of radiocontrast-induced nephropathy. J Am Soc Nephrol 2004; 15: 251–60.

64. Rhoden E, Teloken C, Lucas M et al. Protective effect of allopurinol in the renal ischemia-reperfusion in uninephrectomized rats. Gen Pharmacol 2000; 35: 189–93.

65. Feitoza CQ, Camara NOS, Pinheiro HS et al. Cyclooxygenase 1 and/or 2 blockade ameliorates the renal tissue damage triggered by ischemia and reperfusion injury. Int Immunopharmacol 2005; 5: 79–84.

6

Open nephron-sparing surgery for renal cell carcinoma

Bruce R Kava

INTRODUCTION

Radical nephrectomy is widely accepted as the surgical standard for treatment of renal cell carcinoma. A number of factors, however, have contributed to the increased utilization of nephron-sparing surgery (NSS) in select patients with renal cell carcinoma over the last two decades. The widespread application of diagnostic imaging has resulted in a precipitous increase in the number of incidentally detected renal tumors in North America and Europe.[1,2] Data from the National Cancer Institute's Surveillance Epidemiology and End Results (SEER) program, has demonstrated that localized tumors comprise the majority of these incidentally detected renal tumors, and that this has impacted all age and racial groups.[3]

The increased detection of incidental, asymptomatic tumors has concomitantly resulted in an overall decrease in the average tumor size and stage[1,4–10] over the last 20 years. Herr[7] found, in his single surgeon series, that the average tumor size in patients undergoing surgery for renal cell carcinoma declined from greater than 5 cm to just above 2.5 cm between 1985 and 1996. In another report from the same institution that assessed the experience of several surgeons, the average renal mass decreased in size by 32%, from 7.8 cm to 5.3 cm at approximately the same time interval.[10] Other reports have validated this size and stage migration,[8,9] which has translated into increased utilization of NSS,[7] as well as an overall improvement in disease-free and overall survival.[6]

INDICATIONS FOR NEPHRON-SPARING SURGERY

The indications for NSS have been classified into one of three categories:[11]

1. *Absolute or imperative indications* are those situations in which the patient would be rendered functionally anephric if a radical nephrectomy were performed. Renal cell carcinoma involving an anatomically or functionally solitary kidney and bilateral synchronous renal tumors are specific situations which would fall into this category.

2. *Relative indications* for undergoing NSS are situations in which there exists a unilateral solid renal mass and the contralateral kidney is at risk for future decline in function as a result of another disease or disorder. This would encompass a variety of situations, including: calculus disease, chronic pyelonephritis, renal artery stenosis, diabetes mellitus, and nephrosclerosis.[12] Less common diseases such as vesicoureteral reflux, chronic pyelonephritis, and ureteropelvic junction obstruction may also be considered relative indications for partial nephrectomy. Finally, von Hippel–Lindau disease and other genetic disorders that predispose an individual to the development of a contralateral tumor would be considered a relative indication for partial nephrectomy.

3. *Elective indications* for partial nephrectomy are those situations in which a tumor exists in one kidney and there is a functionally normal contralateral kidney. While the advantages of NSS are clear-cut in patients who would be rendered functionally anephric following radical nephrectomy, elective indications for performing a partial nephrectomy have been utilized increasingly over the last 15 years. The rationale for nephron preservation in these individuals results from (1) the comparable safety and oncologic efficacy of partial nephrectomy when compared with radical nephrectomy for similar stage tumors (see below), (2) the fact that many patients diagnosed with renal cell carcinoma are younger and have years at risk for future decline in

renal function as a result of senescence or competing comorbidites, (3) the relative uncertainty associated with an increased incidence of proteinuria in patients who undergo unilateral nephrectomy,[13] and (4) the increasing recognition of a genetic predisposition for many patients with renal cell carcinoma, in whom metachronous development of a tumor in the remaining renal parenchyma is of concern.

CATEGORIES OF NEPHRON-SPARING SURGERY

The basic surgical principles of partial nephrectomy include (1) mobilization of the kidney with early vascular control, (2) avoidance of prolonged renal ischemia, (3) complete tumor excision with negative surgical margins, (4) closure of the collecting system, and (5) careful hemostasis and closure of the renal defect.[14] Five specific categories of NSS have been described.

Simple tumor enucleation. Many renal tumors are completely surrounded by a distinct pseudocapsule of fibrous tissue.[15] Traditionally, tumor enucleation implies that by bluntly dissecting between the pseudocapsule and the normal renal parenchyma the tumor can be removed with maximal preservation of renal parenchyma. This often can be accomplished without the need for hilar clamping, and hemostasis is usually accomplished quite easily by suture ligation of small peripheral arteries with absorbable suture material.

Several studies have voiced concerns regarding residual microscopic tumor or nests of tumor cells that may exist just beyond the pseudocapsule in patients with renal tumors.[16-19] This raises some doubt regarding the oncologic efficacy of simple tumor enucleation. Some investigators have recommended that a 1 cm tumor-free margin be obtained in order to avoid the 5% incidence of peritumoral satellite lesions that may lead to a local recurrence.[19] Others have argued that the significance of peritumoral satellites is minimal, and that even in the face of microscopically positive margins, the relative risk of local tumor recurrence is extremely low.[20] While still evoking controversy, simple enucleation of renal tumors without confirming tumor-free surgical margins has a very limited role. We recommend that a small amount of healthy, tumor-free renal tissue beyond the pseudocapsule should be excised with the specimen, providing for tumor-free surgical margins. The application of the argon beam coagulator may also provide another 2–3 mm safety margin of tissue necrosis deep to the tumor bed.[7]

Polar segmental nephrectomy, wedge resection, and major transverse resection (Figures 6.1–6.3). The underlying goal of each of these techniques involves mobilization

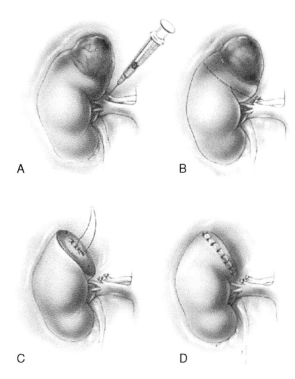

A   B

C   D

Figure 6.1 Polar segmental nephrectomy is performed by first delineating the region within the vascular supply of one of the segmental renal arteries. A margin of healthy renal parenchyma is excised in addition to the tumor. Once hemostasis is achieved and the collecting system is closed, the capsule is reapproximated.

of the kidney within Gerota's fascia, leaving a generous amount of perinephric fat and Gerota's fascia overlying the tumor. The renal hilum is exposed. For polar segmental nephrectomy and major transverse resections, prospective identification and ligation of the segmental arterial supply to the specific tumor-bearing area of the kidney is performed. Injection of methylene blue directly into a segmental artery may outline the limits of the involved renal segment, if there is any uncertainty. For wedge resections, it is not usually necessary to identify the actual segmental branch, as these tumors are usually located in the peripheral regions of the kidney. Prospective identification and suture ligation of small peripheral arteries is accomplished directly as the tumor-bearing region is being excised. This usually occurs after surface hypothermia and hilar clamping. A knowledge of the renal vascular supply is important even in these cases, in order to avoid direct injury to one of the segmental vessels during dissection of the renal hilum.

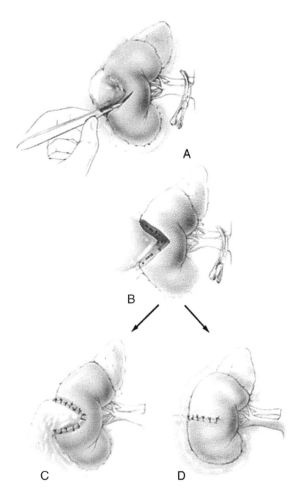

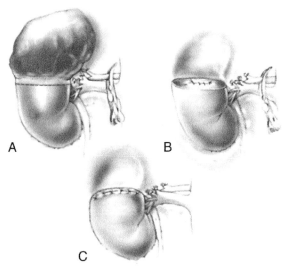

Figure 6.3 Major transverse resection is performed by prospectively identifying and dividing the segmental artery or arteries supplying a major portion of the kidney. A major portion of the kidney is excised with the tumor and the collecting system is reapproximated. Hemostasis is achieved.

Figure 6.2 Wedge resection is performed by circumscribing the tumor with a margin of healthy renal parenchyma. The tumor-containing area is excised with the knife handle, hemostasis is achieved and a small amount of perinephric fat or oxidized cellulose is packed into the tumor bed. The renal capsule is then reapproximated over the area.

Extracorporeal partial nephrectomy with autotransplantation (Figure 6.4) can be utilized for large or multiple complex tumors involving the renal hilum, or for situations in which complex reconstruction of the kidney or renal artery is needed in addition to tumor resection.[21] Generally, extracorporeal surgery is reserved for desperation situations as described above, is not usually advocated for elective nephron sparing surgery, and is not usually necessary for removal of most centrally located tumors.[22] Complications occur in 31–87% of cases, often translating into the need for secondary surgery.[23,24] In one series,[24] a 19% local recurrence rate

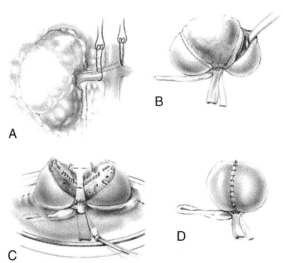

Figure 6.4 Extracorporeal partial nephrectomy with autotransplantation is performed for desperate situations in which there is no other alternative for maintaining adequate renal function in the face of a renal tumor. The complication rate is high and cure rates are less than in situ surgery.

was noted in 16 patients undergoing ex vivo surgery versus 6.1% of the 82 patients undergoing intracorporeal surgery.

An alternative to extracorporeal surgery for select patients with large or multiple complex tumors involving the renal hilum has been suggested by Steffens et al.[25] In this technique, the renal artery and vein are clamped. The renal artery is cannulated and perfused with 500 ml cooled (4°C) Ringer's lactate. Drainage of the perfusate occurs through a small venotomy in the renal vein, on the right. On the left, the perfusate is drained through the divided gonadal vein. Once the perfusate is clear, the arteriotomy in the renal artery is closed. The renal vein is closed on the right, and if the gonadal vein was used, it is ligated. In their series of 65 patients, the mean operative blood loss was 210 ml, there were no vascular reperfusion problems, and only 2 patients with pre-existing anemia required transfusion. Even the most central tumors were resected in a bloodless field, although there were 12 patients (19%) who developed postoperative hemorrhage and 5 (8%) required re-exploration. This is well above the rate reported by most series evaluating NSS. It is unclear why so many patients developed postoperative hemorrhage, and also whether this could be corrected with more meticulous intraoperative hemostasis.

PREOPERATIVE CONSIDERATIONS

A detailed history and physical examination are essential in all patients undergoing NSS. Medical and cardiology clearance are based upon patient age, comorbidities, and perioperative risk factors. There is no substitute for prudent medical judgement. A basic laboratory evaluation is performed, and includes a CBC, serum creatinine determination, liver function tests, coagulation profile, and a urinalysis. The urinalysis should test for the presence of proteinuria. The basic diagnostic imaging that is required is a CT or MRI of the abdomen and pelvis with and without intravenous contrast enhancement, in addition to a chest X-ray. Additional staging imaging studies are based upon the judgement of the physician.

A full discussion of the radiologic imaging of renal tumors is provided elsewhere in this text. Nevertheless, the performance of a partial nephrectomy is in many ways much more challenging than radical nephrectomy. It behooves the surgeon to have a very detailed understanding of the renal and vascular anatomy in order to avoid complications. There is no substitute for a high-quality CT scan or MRI without and with the administration of intravenous contrast. This provides an overall characterization of the size and location of the tumor,

as well as its relationship to the major vascular structures. It provides detail regarding anatomic abnormalities, not only involving the ipsilateral kidney (i.e. accessory renal vessels), but also provides for additional staging information that would argue against partial nephrectomy (i.e. renal vein or inferior vena cava thrombus, lymphadenopathy, or the presence of more advanced, invasive disease). It also provides for an assessment of tumor multifocality.

The use of three-dimensional volume-rendered CT imaging has proven to be extremely accurate in delineating the renal parenchyma and vascular anatomy associated with NSS.[26–28] When available, this is a very useful adjunct to the standard studies and provides an extremely helpful road map for the vascular structures. This is particularly important prior to resecting centrally located tumors.

TECHNIQUE

Positioning the patient undergoing nephron-sparing surgery

An extraperitoneal flank incision is recommended for NSS. While a transperitoneal approach may be utilized for many types of renal surgery, the flank incision is advantageous in that it allows for delivery of any aspect of the kidney to the surface of the wound. Some have recommended an incision through the bed of the 11th or 12th rib,[11,29] although we favor a supracostal incision. This provides excellent exposure to the kidney and adrenal gland, even for large upper pole tumors. We usually utilize the 11th rib, however a supra 12th rib incision may also suffice.

For central tumors or in situations in which there is a high likelihood that the collecting system will be entered, a 5 Fr Pollack catheter may be placed endoscopically into the renal pelvis of the affected kidney. Cystoscopy is performed, with the use of a C-arm fluoroscopy unit, in order to confirm position of the stent. This is performed just prior to positioning the patient for the incision. The presence of a Pollack catheter allows for administration of indigo carmine directly into the collecting system following tumor excision. This facilitates direct visualization of the edges of the collecting system, which can then be closed in an anatomic, and watertight fashion. An alternative technique that may be used is the direct administration of a dilute solution of methylene blue into the renal pelvis with a small 25 gauge needle, after temporary occlusion of the ureter with a vessel loop.[30]

A Foley catheter is placed prior to positioning the patient who is then placed in the standard flank position.

The kidney rest is raised between the contralateral 12th rib and the iliac crest. The table is flexed, and the patient is then positioned in a mild Trendelenburg position (Figure 6.5). The upper leg is extended and the lower leg is flexed. This increases the space between the costal margin and the iliac crest, and puts the flank muscles and skin on tension.[31] A pillow is placed between the two legs and an axillary roll is placed just below the axilla in order to prevent pressure on the brachial plexus. Additional pressure points are identified and well padded. A double arm board or Krauss arm support system is used to support the upper arm. The patient is secured to the table with wide cloth tape that is run over the greater trochanter. A second strip of tape is run over the upper shoulder and is secured to the double arm board anteriorly and the table posteriorly.

Positioning of the patient for NSS is extremely important and it is crucial to work closely with the anesthesia team, as the position may not be tolerated by all patients. Elderly patients and those with diminished cardiac function may not tolerate the impaired venous return caused by the pressure of the kidney rest on the inferior vena cava. In addition, flexion of the table may also contribute to diminishing the return of venous blood from the lower extremities. These ultimately may lead to a decreased cardiac output and systemic hypotension. Liberal hydration, less pronounced positioning, reducing the amount of pressure caused by the kidney rest, and limiting the amount of time that the patient spends in the flank position may be utilized to counteract these effects.

Incision

The patient is rigorously hydrated and mannitol 12.5 g is made available to the anesthesia team for administration 10 minutes prior to clamping the renal artery. For a supracostal 11th rib incision, a skin incision is made precisely over the body of the 11th rib. This extends over the entire course of the rib, from the anterior to the posterior axillary line. If needed, additional exposure can be obtained by extending the incision anteriorly, towards the rectus sheath.

Once the skin and superficial fascia are opened, the latissimus dorsi and the serratus posterior inferior muscles are transected with electrocautery (Figure 6.6). This exposes the entire lateral belly of the 11th rib. The dissection proceeds anteriorly to the rib tip, where the superficial fascia as well as the external and internal oblique muscles are transected using electrocautery. Once the rib is fully exposed, the external intercostal muscle is gently dissected from the upper margin of the rib using electrocautery. We continue to dissect off the external intercostal muscle, following the border of the upper surface of the rib, towards the posterior axillary line. The periosteal elevator is then insinuated directly under the periosteum of the rib (Figure 6.7). By gently elevating the rib, the periosteal elevator is used to dissect the internal intercostal muscle off of the rib, exposing the extrapleural fascia. We proceed in a direction from the rib tip to the posterior axillary line. Great care must be taken during the posterior portion of the dissection in order to avoid inadvertent injury to the pleura. Just prior to dissecting the pleura and diaphragm off of the rib,

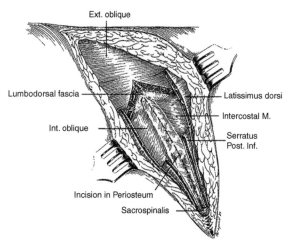

Figure 6.6 A supracostal incision is made. The incision is made directly over the rib. The latissimus dorsi and serratus posterior inferior muscles are divided. Anteriorly the external oblique and internal oblique muscles are divided. Great care is used in avoidance of inadvertent injury to the intercostal nerves.

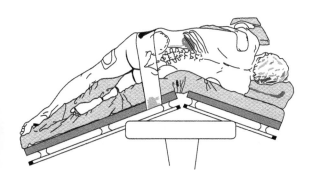

Figure 6.5 Standard flank positioning. The patient is well padded, the lower leg flexed, while the upper leg is extended. A bean bag is placed in order to maintain stability and the kidney rest is elevated. An axillary roll must be placed and all pressure points are padded.

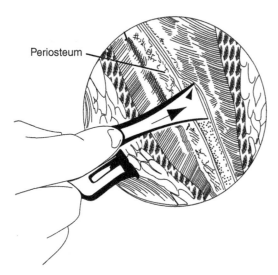

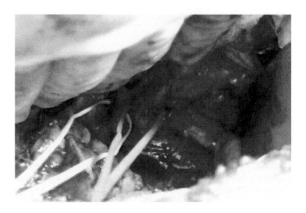

Figure 6.8 Renal hilar control is obtained by placing vessel loops around the renal artery (blue loop) and the renal vein (red loop).

Figure 6.7 The periosteal elevator is insinuated under the periosteum of the rib. It is used to develop a plane between the rib and the underlying extrapleural fascia, in order to prevent injury to the pleura.

we find it helpful to incise the lumbodorsal fascia, which can be found just under the rib tip. The peritoneum is swept anteriorly and the remaining layers of the abdominal wall (internal oblique and transversus abdominus muscles) are opened. The intercostal nerve exits from under the lower border of the rib, and great care must be taken to identify this structure between the internal oblique and transversus muscles.

Once the lumbodorsal fascia is opened, Gerota's fascia can be seen. A plane is developed between the posterior leaf of Gerota's fascia and the psoas fascia. This allows for a three-dimensional visualization of the diaphragm and its attachments into the lower ribs. These attachments are sharply and carefully taken down to allow for upward deflection of the pleura and full visualization of the intercostal nerve. If an inadvertent pleurotomy is made, it can usually be closed later, at the time of wound closure.

At this time, the costovertebral ligaments are divided from the upper margin of the posterior aspect of the rib. The release of these ligaments allows for easy downward deflection of the rib, similar to the handle of a bucket.

Mobilization of the kidney

Gerota's fascia is mobilized and dissected off of the psoas fascia postero-medially. The ureter and either the vena cava or aorta are identified at the infero-medial aspect of the dissection. The ureter is used as a landmark, and the peritoneal reflection is then dissected off

of the anterior surface of Gerota's fascia, proceeding superiorly and laterally. The ureter is tagged with a vessel loop, which facilitates its identification later. The gonadal vein can usually be found just lateral to the ureter and usually crosses the ureter anteriorly as it proceeds to enter into the inferior vena cava (on the right) or the left renal vein. It can be preserved or, if further dissection is needed, may be ligated.

When operating on the right kidney, the duodenum is mobilized using the Kocher maneuver. The renal hilum is identified. Both the renal artery and renal vein are fully mobilized. On the left side, great care is taken in order to avoid injury to the gonadal and adrenal branches of the renal vein. All major vessels should be carefully identified and tagged with vessel loops (Figure 6.8).

The remainder of the attachments of Gerota's fascia are freed superiorly at this time and mannitol 12.5 g is administered intravenously by the anesthesia team. Gerota's fascia is opened at a site that is situated well away from the tumor. The kidney surface is identified and dissection is performed with great care to allow for preservation of an intact renal capsule. If an inadvertent capsulotomy is made, readjustment is needed in order to avoid denuding a large area of capsule that will be predisposed to bleeding. The area around the tumor is identified and Gerota's fascia is left intact over this area. Once the region around the tumor is identified it is now time for administration of surface hypothermia.

Administration of surface hypothermia

Traditionally it has been thought that warm ischemia times longer than 30 minutes are detrimental to the aerobic metabolism of the kidney. Subsequently, renal hypothermia is established after hilar clamping in those cases in which the duration of warm ischemia is anticipated to exceed 30 minutes. Renal hypothermia induces short-term suspension of renal metabolism, provides cellular protection, and minimizes postischemic renal injury in patients undergoing partial nephrectomy.[32] Surface cooling of the kidney allows for as much as 3 hours of safe ischemic time, and is not thought to induce irreversible insult to the kidney.[33]

A bowel bag can be placed around the outside of Gerota's fascia, leaving the renal vessels exposed (Figure 6.8). A vascular clamp is placed on the renal artery and ice slush is packed around the exposed kidney within the bowel bag. For larger, more centrally located tumors a clamp is also placed on the renal vein. This limits the amount of venous back-bleeding during these more complicated surgeries.

Surface hypothermia is maintained for 10 minutes, in order to decrease core temperature to 15 to 20°C before commencing tumor resection.[11] Once this time period has elapsed, the electrocautery is used to make a circumferential incision extending just through the renal capsule, approximately 1 cm around the renal tumor. For those intrarenal tumors that are not readily palpable, intraoperative ultrasonography has been used (Figures 6.9–6.11) in order to identify the location,[34] as well as the topographic extent of deep tumors.[35] It also may help to define tumor proximity to vascular structures.[36,37] One study suggested that intraoperative ultrasound was helpful in identifying previously unrecognized tumors in cases of multifocal tumors.[38] However, a prospective study found that intraoperative ultrasonography offered no advantage to preoperative CT and intraoperative assessment in determining the presence of additional occult renal tumors.[39]

Once the renal capsule is incised, the blunt end of a knife handle is used to gently develop a plane that excises the tumor with a small amount of normal appearing parenchyma around it. As the dissection continues medially, larger renal segmental arterial branches can usually be prospectively identified and suture ligated prior to transecting them. This avoids retraction of these vessels into the surrounding parenchyma, which makes later identification difficult. We use 2/0 or 3/0 monocril

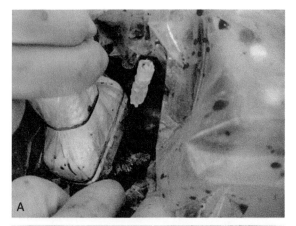

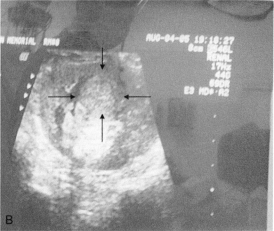

Figure 6.10 Intraoperative ultrasound is performed for a tumor that is impalpable. A spinal needle is used to identify the area in which the tumor is present (A). The depth of the tumor and its location can be determined by the interference pattern that the spinal needle causes on the ultrasound image. The tumor (B) is seen within the arrows.

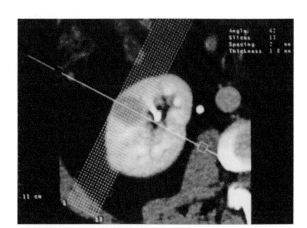

Figure 6.9 A centrally located tumor that has no exophytic component to it. Identification of these tumors is made possible by the use of intraoperative ultrasonography. The line that is perpendicular to the long axis of the kidney approximates the angle in which intraoperative ultrasound would confirm the most direct route in which to approach this tumor.

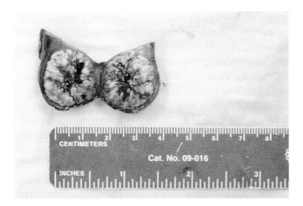

Figure 6.11 The tumor (yellow) was identified and was excised with a rim of healthy (darker brown) renal parenchyma.

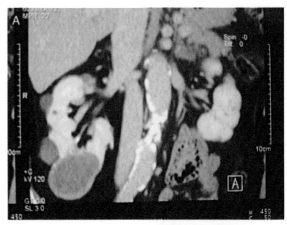

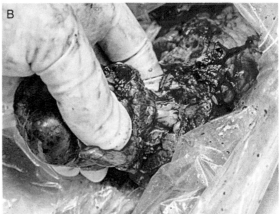

Figure 6.12 This complex renal cyst has a thickened wall (indicated by arrows), which enhances with intravenous contrast (A). A segmental polar nephrectomy was performed. The lower pole of the kidney with a rim of normal, healthy tissue is excised with the tumor (B). For illustration, the perinephric fat and Gerota's fascia were removed.

(monofilament poliglecaprone 25) or chromic suture material with a UR-6 needle for suture ligation of these small arteries. The tight curvature of these needles allows for ligation of small vessels, without incorporating a large amount of the adjacent normal renal parenchyma. In addition, by using monocril or chromic catgut, the suture material slides through the renal parenchyma without causing too much shearing and fraying of the renal parenchyma. Tying down the knots of these sutures requires practice, as overzealous tying of the suture material tends to rip entirely through the renal parenchyma.

Once the tumor has been completely excised, random biopsies of the renal parenchyma that exist within the crater that has been produced are sent for frozen section analysis. Visual inspection of the tumor-bearing tissue may be helpful in identifying areas in which there is a paucity of normal renal parenchyma around the tumor. If this is the case, the decision to perform a deeper partial nephrectomy or to remove the entire kidney will depend upon the judgement of the operating surgeon.

While waiting for the frozen sections to be processed, careful suture ligation of small peripheral vessels that are noted within the tumor bed is performed. If a vascular clamp was used on the renal vein it should be removed and hyperinflation of the lungs by the anesthesia team can be used in order to enhance visualization of the venous system. The collecting system can be assessed by instillation of indigo carmine through the Pollack catheter, if it was placed. If open, the collecting system is reapproximated with 20 or 30 chromic catgut or 30 monocryl suture material (Figures 6.12 and 6.13). A water-tight closure of the collecting system is highly desirable and can be tested by additional instillation of indigo carmine or methylene blue through the Pollack catheter.

Once tumor-free margins have been confirmed, coagulation of the base of the tumor is then performed. The argon beam coagulator can then be applied to the surface of the tumor bed, providing for an additional 2–3 mm of coagulative necrosis. Overzealous use of coagulation current over the suture material or the collecting system should be avoided, as it may weaken or completely disrupt the suture material that was placed.

Closure of the tumor bed

Once hemostasis has been confirmed and the collecting system has been closed, there are a variety of agents that can be used over the surface of the tumor bed,

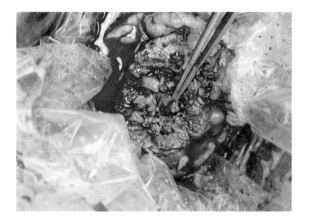

Figure 6.13 Following polar segmental nephrectomy for a deeply penetrating tumor, the collecting system was reapproximated with 2/0 absorbable monocril suture material. It is seen very well here, following administration of indigo carmine or methylene blue through a previously placed Pollack catheter.

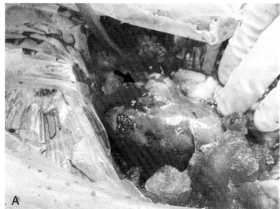

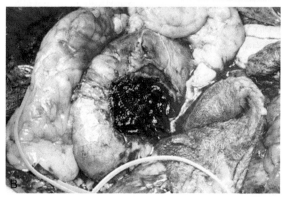

Figure 6.14 A wedge resection was performed for this renal tumor (A). A bowel bag was placed around the kidney and surface hypothermia was administered, as can be seen by the ice slush around the kidney. For illustration purposes, the perinephric fat has been removed from around the mass. The tumor was excised and, after negative frozen sections were confirmed, the argon beam coagulator was used for hemostasis. Oxidized cellulose was stuffed into the tumor bed (B) and it was later closed with liver sutures.

prior to unclamping the artery. Fibrin sealants have been found to be quite helpful,[40–42] but are not a substitute for meticulous hemostasis. We have found that a gelatin matrix thrombin tissue sealant (Floseal) is very helpful in obtaining rapid hemostasis following partial nephrectomy. Application of this agent to the resection bed while the renal artery is still clamped provides excellent hemostasis within 1–2 minutes.[43,44] The base is then packed with a hemostatic agent, such as oxidized cellulose (Figure 6.14). Once this is in place, we place liver sutures (0 chromic) using blunt tip needles in a horizontal mattress closure of the renal parenchyma and capsule. These sutures are placed through the capsule to a depth of approximately one-third of the way down through the parenchyma. Gel foam bolsters are used to prevent the knots of the liver sutures from ripping through the renal parenchyma.

Once the capsule has been reapproximated the renal artery is unclamped and the kidney is watched to insure reperfusion. Occasionally the artery may still be kinked and it may also develop transient arterial spasm. We reapproximate the kidney into its normal preoperative position. If needed, a nephropexy may be performed in order to insure that the ureter does not kink after a portion of the kidney is removed. If bleeding is noted, the vascular clamp is reapplied and the closure is taken down to inspect the area of the tumor bed. Once reperfusion and hemostasis have been confirmed, the preserved perirenal fat is then secured over the suture line of the renal parenchyma and Gerota's fascia is reapproximated. If there is a paucity of retained perirenal fat or Gerota's fascia, the peritoneal edge may be used for this purpose. A Jackson Pratt drain is placed along the psoas fascia, in a dependent position. We attempt to provide some separation of the drain and the kidney, as placing the closed suction drain too close to the collecting system may promote a urinary fisula. Others use a Penrose drain.[11]

At the time of the abdominal closure the vessel loops are removed. If the pleura needs to be closed, a red rubber catheter is placed into the chest. 20 silk or vicryl suture material is used to close the pleura in a running fashion. Just prior to tying the suture down, the chest is insufflated while the red rubber catheter is placed under water seal. After several deep inspiratory efforts administered by the anesthesia team, the red rubber catheter is slowly backed out of the pleural space, while remaining under water seal. Once it is removed, the knot is tied. If any doubt regarding a persistent pneumothorax exists, an upright chest X-ray is obtained in the operating room, where a formal chest tube may be placed if needed.

The drain is secured to the skin and the wound is closed in two layers. Closure of a flank incision needs to be performed carefully. Care must be exerted in avoiding inadvertent injury to the pleura, as well as in avoiding incorporation of the intercostal nerve bundle in the closure. A two-layered closure is advocated: the first layer incorporates the transversus abdominus and internal oblique muscles and fascia, the second layer incorporates the external oblique muscle and fascia. Posteriorly, the external intercostal muscles are reappoximated, and the latissimus dorsi and the serratus posterior inferior are reapproximated in separate layers.

POSTOPERATIVE CARE

The patient undergoing partial nephrectomy should be given liberal amounts of intravenous fluids, if possible during the first 24 hours. The use of sequential compression devices, encouraging early ambulation, and the use of respiratory inspirometry are extremely important adjuncts in preventing early complications such as atalectasis and thromboembolic events. With the application of these principles, we have not found a need for systemic anticoagulation, which carries the risk for postoperative bleeding. Most patients are started immediately on a clear liquid diet, and may be advanced to a regular diet as tolerated. The Foley catheter is usually left in place until the patient is ambulating without assistance, usually at 48 hours. Once the patient is tolerating a diet, ambulating, and the incisional pain is well controlled with oral agents, they may be discharged home. Antibiotics are usually not administered for more than 24–48 hours perioperatively. If a stent was placed, it is usually removed 4–6 weeks postoperatively.

COMPLICATIONS OF NEPHRON-SPARING SURGERY

Complications of NSS consist of those that are relatively non-specific and those that are procedure-specific. Table 6.1 outlines the major complications which occurred in 3.2–37% of patients from several contemporary series of patients undergoing NSS.[10,23,24,45–52]

The wide variability in complication rates reflects the heterogeneity of the patients within the various series. Age, operative time, and pathologic stage have all been found to be independently associated with a higher risk for early complications following NSS.[51] Interestingly, one surgeon in this multivariate analysis had a significantly greater number of perioperative complications, even when controling for other perioperative risk factors. This underscores the need for attention to detail, especially with regard to hemostasis and a water-tight closure of the collecting system.

As more elective NSS is performed, and as experience grows with these techniques,[23,30] the complication rate will undoubtedly continue to decline. In the series reported by Campbell et al,[23] incidentally discovered tumors had fewer complications than those that were symptomatic. However, the 50% reduction in complications associated with NSS in patients even with symptomatic tumors between 1989 and 1994 could only reflect improvements in surgical technique as well as better selection of patients for NSS. Finally, in both the series by Lerner et al[24] and Campbell et al,[23] extracorporeal surgery was associated with significantly higher overall complication rates than intracorporeal surgery.

Perioperative mortality is extremely low following NSS. Of the 10 perioperative deaths listed in Table 6.1, three patients died of perioperative cardiac complications, three died of sepsis, and one each died from pneumonia, a ruptured thoracic aortic aneurysm, and a renal vein thrombus requiring emergent thrombectomy. In one series, the cause of death was not indicated.[30] Of note, 5 of the 10 reported deaths were precipitated by perioperative hemorrhage and 4 of the perioperative deaths were preceded by reoperation.

Postoperative urinary fistula occurs in 0–17.4% of patients. Campbell et al[23] defined a fistula as persistent drainage of >50 ml per day with an elevated (greater than 2.0) drainage fluid to serum creatinine ratio. They found an increased risk for fistula in patients with centrally located tumors, the need for major reconstruction of the collecting system, tumors >4 cm, and for patients undergoing extracorporeal surgery with autotransplantation.

Not all patients who develop fistulae require ureteral stent placement. In fact, of the 12 series in which 95 fistulas were reported, only 26 (27%) were actually treated with a ureteral stent placement. Management of all of the fistulas reported by Polascik et al[30] was expectant, with the exception of one patient requiring percutaneous drainage of a urinoma. Median time to fistula closure was 46 days in 20 patients reported by Stephenson et al,[51] and only 4 patients (1.1%) required a ureteral stent placement for resolution.

Table 6.1 Major complications and their incidence in several contemporary series of patients undergoing nephron-sparing surgery

Series	n	% Imperative	Overall complications (%)	Hemorrhage	Fistula	OR for stent	Acute renal failure (%)/requiring permanent dialysis (%)	Number requiring secondary surgery (%)	Perioperative mortality
Campbell et al 1994[23]	259	96	78 (30)	6 (2.3)	45 (17.4)	14 (5)	33 (13)/9 (3)	25 (10)	4 (1.5)
Polascik et al 1995[30]	66	79	25 (37)	1 (1.4)	6 (8.9)	0	NI	1 (1.4)	1 (1.4)
Butler et al 1995[45]	46	85	7 (15)	1	3 (6.5)	0	1 (2)/0	0	1 (2.1)
Lerner et al 1996[24]	185	34	12 (6.4)	0	4	1	NI/2 (1)	6 (3)	1 (0.5)
Duque et al 1998[46]	66	36	18 (27)	3 (4.5)	6 (9.1)	NI	10 (15)/1 (3)	2 (3.1)	0
Belldegrun et al 1999[47]	146	57	8 (5.5)	3 (2)	2 (1.4)	2 (1.4)	NI	5 (3.4)	3 (2)
Lee et al 2000[10]	79	63	9 (11)	0	0	0	0	0	0
Ghavamian et al 2002[48]	63	100	15 (23.8)	1 (1.6)	2 (3.2)	2 (3.2)	8 (12.7)/1 (1.6)	7 (11.1)	0
Shekarriz et al 2002[49]	60	51.6	6 (10)	0	5 (8.3)	1 (1.6)	0	0	0
Adkins et al 2003[50]	30	100	2 (7)	0	0	0	2 (7)**/0	0	0
Stephenson et al 2004[51]	361	19	69 (19)	3 (0.8)	20 (5.5)	4	7 (2)/0	5*	0
Becker et al 2005[52]	311	0	10 (3.2)	8	2	2	0	10	0
University of Miami 2007[†]	94	14	7 (7.4%)	0	0	0	2 (2)/0	0	0

* These two patients had a solitary kidney with already existing renal insufficiency.

** Four patients required interventional radiology.

† Unpublished data.

There has been a generalized decline in the incidence of fistulae, with more contemporary series reporting a lower incidence. This decline likely reflects a greater number of elective cases of NSS, as well as more meticulous identification and closure of the collecting system. In fact, Polacek et al[30] reported that all of the fistulae in their series occurred prior to 1988. It was at that time that they began to delineate the collecting system with methylene blue instillation.

Acute renal failure (ARF) following partial nephrectomy occurs in 2–13% of cases, and is much more common in patients who have imperative indications for partial nephrectomy. It is thought to arise from a combination of intraoperative ischemia and removal of functional renal parenchyma during NSS. Less commonly, it may result from relatively non-specific reasons such as inadequate perioperative fluid resuscitation, drug interactions, or sepsis. Campbell et al[23] found that ARF occurred in 26% of 115 patients undergoing partial nephrectomy in a solitary kidney, compared with an incidence of 2% in 144 patients with a contralateral kidney. In addition, ARF was more likely to occur in patients with tumors >7 cm, patients undergoing excision of >50% of the renal parenchyma, and for ischemic times >60 minutes. Despite this, ARF resolves spontaneously in the majority of patients following NSS. The need for permanent dialysis occurs in less than 3% of cases, and is also undoubtedly associated with the amount of preserved renal parenchyma.

Postoperative bleeding following partial nephrectomy occurs in less than 2% of most contemporary cohorts. Although several older series have reported significant re-exploration rates in the event of postoperative hemorrhage, Stevenson et al[51] indicated that the majority of patients who develop postoperative hemorrhage can be managed conservatively or with angioembolization.

In older series, the *average length of stay* following NSS was between 7 and 9 days.[45,53,54] In more contemporary series the average length of stay has diminished to 5–6.4 days.[50,51] In one series, a reduction in the length of stay to 4 days was achieved by utilizing a clinical pathway system which emphasized perioperative teaching, encouraged early ambulation, and provided optimal pain management.[50] Part of the impetus for this reduction in the average length of stay has been attributed to diminished complications, which ultimately translates into a reduction in overall hospital costs.[54]

TRANSFUSION RATES ASSOCIATED WITH NEPHRON-SPARING SURGERY

There has been some variability in the reported blood loss and transfusion rates in patients undergoing NSS.

Blood loss appears to be higher in patients with imperative indications for NSS. In a series of 66 patients undergoing NSS, Duque et al[46] reported that the mean blood loss was 1127 ml (range 200–3200 ml) in patients with a solitary kidney vs 402 ml (range 100–1200 ml) in patients with elective indications. Moreover, 86% of patients with a solitary kidney required perioperative transfusion versus 17% of those undergoing NSS with a normal contralateral kidney. In a retrospective review of all patients undergoing kidney cancer surgery at one institution, Shvarts et al[55] also found that blood loss in NSS exceeded that of patients undergoing radical nephrectomy, with 30% of these patients receiving blood transfusions. As mentioned above, NSS for centrally situated tumors may be technically challenging, and also may be associated with a high risk of excessive blood loss and subsequent transfusion of blood products. Drachenberg et al[56] reported a mean transfusion requirement of 6.7 units of blood during 44 partial nephrectomies performed for centrally located tumors. Overall, 32 (73%) of the 44 patients in their series required at least one unit of transfused blood.

Several groups, however, have found no difference in the requirements for blood transfusion in patients undergoing NSS compared with those undergoing radical nephrectomy.[44,49,52] Curiously, 15–30% of patients in these series underwent blood transfusions despite reasonably low amounts of reported blood loss. These high transfusion rates may reflect underestimation of blood loss associated with the procedures, or preoperative anemia resulting from chronic illness or renal insufficiency, or it may be that these centers have taken a more liberal attitude to the administration of blood products. In dramatic contrast to this, in one recent series of 30 patients undergoing NSS for imperative indications, only one patient (3%) received a transfusion in the perioperative period.[48] Similarly, less than 5% of patients at our center have undergone perioperative transfusions (unpublished data).

ONCOLOGIC EFFICACY AND COMPARISON OF NEPHRON-SPARING SURGERY WITH RADICAL NEPHRECTOMY

NSS offers high cure rates for select patients with renal cell carcinoma. Table 6.2 lists a number of studies that have reported long-term follow-up for patients undergoing NSS for renal cell carcinoma. What has become apparent as these studies have matured is that patients undergoing primarily elective NSS[7,52] and those patients with tumors measuring 4 cm or less[10,24,47,57,58] represent a group of patients with long-term success rates approaching 100%.

Table 6.2 Results for contemporary series of patients undergoing nephron sparing surgery

Series	n	% Elective	Follow-up (months)	Mean tumor size (cm)	Cancer specific survival		Local only (%)	Recurrence (%) local + distant	Distant only
					5-year	10-year			
Ghavamian et al 2002[48]	63	0	76.8	4	81	64	7 (11)	0	21 (33)
Steffans et al 2005[25]	65	0	95	NI	76	76	0	0	14 (22)
Hafez et al 1999[57]	485	9	47	2.7	92	80	7 (1.4)	9 (1.8)	28 (5.8)
Fergany et al 2000[58]	107	10	104	NI	88	73	4 (4)	7 (6.5)	23 (21.5)
Lerner et al 1996[24]	185	34	44	4.1	89	77	11 (5.9)*	NS	NS
Belldegrun et al 1999[47]	146	43	74	3.6	91	NI	4 (2.7)	0	8 (5.5)
Lee et al 2000[10]	79	47	40	2.5	95	NI	0	0	3 (4)
Herr 1999[7]	70	100	120	3	97	97	0	1 (1.5)	1 (1.5)
Becker et al 2006[52]	241	100	66	3.7	98	96	3 (1.4)	0	9 (4.2)

* Indicates that only 25–30 month follow-up was obtained instead of the 5-year disease-free survival reported for the other series.

Table 6.3 Comparison of radical nephrectomy with nephron-sparing surgery. A number of contemporary series have compared complication rates and oncologic outcome in patients undergoing nephron-sparing surgery with matched controls undergoing radical nephrectomy

Series	Treatment (n)	Complications (%)	5-Year DFS (%)	Selection criteria for matched controls
Butler et al 1995[45]	RN (42)	6 (14)	8.5	Matched for date of surgery, all tumors <4 cm
	PN (46)	7 (15)	9.2	
Lerner et al 1996[24]	RN (209)	4 (2)	89	Matched for age, sex, date of surgery, tumor location, pathologic stage, and grade
	PN (185)	12 (6.4)	89	
Uzzo et al 1999[54]	RN (28)	2 (7)	96.5*	Matched for date of surgery, all tumors <4 cm
	PN (52)	4 (8)	100	
Belledegrun et al 1999[47]	RN (125)	10 (8)	T1:97/T2:91.4	Matched for age, sex, date of surgery, pathologic stage, and follow-up time
	PN (146)	8 (5.5)	T1:100/T2:66	
Corman et al 2000[53]	RN (1373)	206 (15)	NI	Matched for date of surgery
	PN (512)	83 (16.2)	NI	
Lau et al 2000[60]	RN (164)	10 (6)	98	Matched for age, gender, date of surgery, tumor size, pathologic stage, and grade
	PN (164)	11 (7)	97	
Lee et al 2000[10]	RN (183)	25 (14)	95	Matched for date of surgery, all tumors <4 cm
	PN (79)	9 (11)	95	
Shekarriz et al 2002[49]	RN (60)	2 (3.3)	NI	Matched for age, gender, tumor location and size, and pathologic stage
	PN (60)	6 (10)	NI	
Stephenson et al 2004[51]	RN (688)	112 (16)	NI	Matched for date of surgery
	PN (361)	68 (19)	NI	

* 25–30 month follow-up.

DFS, disease-free survival; RN, radical nephrectomy; PN, partial nephrectomy; NI, not indicated; T1, tumors $\geq$ 2.5 cm (limited to the kidney); T2, tumors >2.5 cm (limited to the kidney).

Although there has been only one small prospective study comparing NSS with radical nephrectomy,[59] both NSS and radical nephrectomy appear to provide equally effective and curative treatment for patients with solitary, small, unilateral renal cell carcinoma. What has likewise become apparent is that they are equally safe. Table 6.3 provides a list of the complications and the 5-year disease-free survival from several series that have compared NSS with matched controls undergoing radical nephrectomy from their respective institutions.

Despite the heterogeneity in patient populations studied, most series have demonstrated that NSS offers a safe and equally effective option for select renal cancers. Cancer-specific survival appears to be more dependent upon tumor stage and histology rather than the type of surgical procedure employed, particularly for those tumors that are 4 cm or less.[10,24,45,47,54] For those patients with T2 lesions, however, Belldegrun et al[47] showed that radical nephrectomy offers a 10-year survival advantage (91.4% vs 66%, $p = 0.001$).

CONCLUSIONS

The dramatic increase in the incidence of incidentally found, small, and localized renal tumors has resulted in an increased utilization of NSS. Indications for NSS include absolute indications, relative indications, and elective indications. The incidence of NSS for elective indications has increased tremendously, fueled by low perioperative morbidity and excellent outcome data generated by many institutions. The technical components of NSS are discussed within the chapter. It is important that the surgeon be meticulous and conscientious in mobilizing the kidney, establishing vascular control, using surface hypothermia when the warm ischemia time is estimated to be more than 30 minutes, maintaining excellent hemostasis, and providing a water-tight closure of the collecting system. Complications may arise following NSS, most do not require additional surgery. However, endoscopic and interventional radiology treatment of these perioperative complications may occasionally be needed.

The short-term complication rate and long-term outcome data for select patients with renal tumors undergoing NSS and radical surgery are comparable. For patients with tumors >4 cm there may be an advantage for radical nephrectomy. However, these risks must be weighed against the risk of renal insufficiency, particularly for those patients with already altered renal function.

REFERENCES

1. Konnak JW, Grossman H. Renal cell carcinoma as an incidental finding. J Urol 1985; 134: 1094–6.

2. Smith SJ, Bosniak MA, Megibow AJ et al. Renal cell carcinoma: earlier discovery and increased detection. Radiology 1989; 170: 699–703.

3. Chow W, Devesa SS, Warrne JL et al. Rising incidence of renal cell cancer in the United States. JAMA 1999; 281: 1628–31.

4. Nakano E, Iwasaki A, Seguchi T et al. Incidentally diagnosed renal cell carcinomas. Eur Urol 1992; 21: 294–8.

5. Thompson IM, Peek M: Improvement in survival of patients with renal cell carcinoma – the role of serendipitously detected tumour. J Urol 1988; 140: 487–90.

6. Sweeney JP, Thornhill JA, Grainger R et al. Incidentally detected renal cell carcinoma: pathological features, survival trends, and implications for treatment. BJU Int 1996; 78: 351–3.

7. Herr HW: Partial nephrectomy for unilateral renal carcinoma and a normal contralateral kidney: 10-year follow up. J Urol 1999; 161: 33–5.

8. Tsui K, Shvarts O, Smith RB et al. Renal cell carcinoma: prognostic significance of incidentally detected tumors. J Urol 2000; 163: 426–30.

9. Luciani LG, Cestari R, Tallarigo C. Incidental renal cell carcinoma – age and stage characterization and clinical implications: study of 1092 patients (1982–1997). Urology 2000; 56: 58–62.

10. Lee CT, Katz J, Shi W et al. Surgical management of renal tumors 4 cm or less in a contemporary cohort. J Urol 2000; 163: 730–6.

11. Uzzo RG, Novick AC. Nephron sparing surgery for renal tumors: indications, techniques, and outcomes. J Urol 2001; 166: 6–18.

12. Licht M, Novick AC. Nephron-sparing surgery for renal cell carcinoma. Urology 1993; 149: 1–7.

13. Selli C, Lapini A, Rizzo M. Conservative surgery of kidney tumors in adults. World J Urol 1992; 10: 30–4.

14. Novick AC. Nephron-sparing surgery for renal cell carcinoma. Annu Rev Med 2002; 53: 393–407.

15. Novick AC. Partial nephrectomy for renal cell carcinoma. Urol Clin North Am 1987; 14: 419–33.

16. Novick AC, Zincke H, Neves RJ et al. Surgical enucleation for renal cell carcinoma. J Urol 1986; 135: 235–8.

17. Marshall FF, Taxy JB, Fishman EK et al. The feasibility of surgical enucleation for renal cell carcinoma. J Urol 1986; 135: 231–4.

18. Blackley SK, Ladaga L, Woolfitt RA et al. Ex situ study of the effectiveness of enucleation in patients with renal cell carcinoma. J Urol 1988; 140: 6–10.

19. Zucchi A, Mearini L, Mearini E et al. Renal cell carcinoma: histological finding on surgical margins after nephron sparing surgery. J Urol 2003; 169: 905–8.

20. Sutherland SE, Resnick MI, MacLennan GT et al. Does the size of surgical margin in partial nephrectomy for renal cell cancer really matter? J Urol 2002; 167: 61–4.

21. Campbell SC, Novick AC, Streem SB et al. Management of renal cell carcinoma with coexistent renal artery disease. J Urol 1993; 150: 808–13.

22. Novick AC, Streem SB, Montie JE et al. Conservative surgery for renal cell carcinoma: a single center experience with 100 cases. J Urol 1989; 141: 835–9.

23. Campbell SC, Novick AC, Streem S et al. Complications of nephron sparing surgery for renal tumors. J Urol 1994; 151: 1177–80.

24. Lerner SE, Hawkins CA, Blute ML et al. Disease outcome in patients with low stage renal cell carcinoma treated with nephron sparing or radical surgery. J Urol 1996; 155: 1868–73.

25. Steffans J, Humke U, Ziegler M et al. Partial nephrectomy with perfusion cooling for imperative indications: a 24-year experience. BJU Int 2005; 96: 608–11.

26. Coll DM, Uzzo RG, Herts BR et al. 3-Dimensional volume rendered computerized tomography for preoperative evaluation and intraoperative treatment of patients undergoing nephron sparing surgery. J Urol 1999; 161: 1097–102.

27. Chernoff DM, Silverman SG, Kikinis R et al. Three-dimensional imaging and display of renal tumors using spiral CT: a potential aid to partial nephrectomy. Urology 1994; 43: 125–9.

28. Wunderlich H, Reichelt O, Schubert R et al. Preoperative simulation of partial nephrectomy with three-dimensional computed tomography. BJU Int 2000; 86: 771–81.

29. Tsui K, van Ophoven A, Shvarts O. Nephron sparing surgery for renal cell carcinioma. Rev Urol 1999; 1(4): 216–25.

30. Polascik TJ, Pound CR, Ment MV et al. Partial nephrectomy: technique, complications, and pathological findings. J Urol 1995; 154: 1312–18.

31. Walsh PC. Surgical approaches to the kidney. In: Medreviews Campbell's Urology, eighth edition. Saunders, 2002.

32. Derweesh IH, Novick AC: Renal ischemia: pathophysiology and clinical impact. AUA Update Series 2006, Lesson 33, Vol 25, 302–7.

33. Novick AC. Renal hypothermia: in vivo and ex vivo. Urol Clin North Am 1983; 10: 637–44.

34. Gilbert BR, Russo P, Zirinski K et al. Intraoperative sonography: application in renal carcinoma. J Urol 1988; 139: 582–4.

35. Assimos DG, Boyce H, Woodruff RD et al. Intraoperative renal ultrasonography: a useful adjunct to partial nephrectomy. J Urol 1991; 146: 1218–20.

36. Walther MM, Choyke PL, Hayes W et al. Evaluation of color Doppler intraoperative ultrasound in parenchymal sparing renal surgery. J Urol 1994; 152: 1984–7.

37. Polascik TJ, Meng MV, Epstein JI et al. Intraoperative sonography for the evaluation and management of renal tumors: experience with 100 patients. J Urol 1995; 154: 1676–80.

38. Marshall FF, Holdford SS, Hamper UM. Intraoperative sonoraphy of renal tumors. J Urol 1992; 148: 1393–6.

39. Campbell SC, Fichtner J, Novick AC et al. Intraoperative evaluation of renal cell carcinoma: a prospective study of the role of ultrasonography and histopathological frozen sections. J Urol 1996; 155: 1191–5.

40. Shekarriz B, Stoller ML. The use of fibrin sealant in urology. J Urol 2002; 67: 1218–25.

41. Janetschek G, Daffner P, Peschel R et al. Laparoscopic nephron sparing surgery for small renal cell carcinoma. J Urol 1998; 159: 1152–5.

42. Levinson AK, Swanson DA, Johnson DE et al. Fibrin glue for partial nephrectomy. Urology 1991; 38: 314–6.

43. Richter F, Schnorr D, Deger S et al. Improvement in hemostasis in open and laparoscopically performed partial nephrectomy using a gelatine matrix-thrombin tissue sealant (Floseal). Urology 2003; 61: 73–7.

44. Richter F, Tullman M, Turk I et al. Gelatine–matrix–thrombin tissue sealant (Floseal) as a tool for effective hemostasis in open and laparoscopic partial nephrectomies. J Urol 2003; 169(Suppl): 22.

45. Butler BP, Novick AC, Miller DP et al. Management of small unilateral renal cell carcinomas: radical versus nephron-sparing surgery. Urol 1995; 45: 34–40.

46. Duque JL, Loughlin KR, O'Leary MP et al. Partial nephrectomy: alternative treatment for selected patients with renal cell carcinoma. Urol 1998; 52: 584–90.

47. Belldegrun A, Tsui K-H, deKernion JB et al. Efficacy of nephron-sparing surgery for renal cell carcinoma: analysis based on the new 1997 tumor-node-metastasis staging system. J Clin Oncol 1999; 17: 2868–75.

48. Ghavamian R, Cheville JC, Lohse CM et al. Renal cell carcinoma in the solitary kidney: an analysis of complications and outome after nephron sparing surgery. J Urol 2002; 168: 454–9.

49. Shekarriz B, Upadhyay J, Shekarriz H et al. Comparison of costs and complications of radical and partial nephrectomy for treatment of localized renal cell carcinoma. Urol 2002; 59: 211–15.

50. Adkins KL, Chang SS, Cookson MS et al. Partial nephrectomy safely preserves renal function in patients with a solitary kidney. J Urol 2003; 169: 79–81.

51. Stephenson AJ, Hakimi A, Snyder ME et al. Complications of radical and partial nephrectomy in a large contemporary cohort. J Urol 2004; 171: 130–4.

52. Becker F, Siemer S, Humke U et al. Elective nephron sparing surgery should become standard treatment for small unilateral renal cell carcinoma: long term survival data of 216 patients. Eur Urol 2006; 49: 308–13.

53. Corman JM, Penson DF, Hur K et al. Comparison of complications after radical and partial nephrectomy: results from the National Veterans Administration Surgical Quality Improvement Program. BJU Int 2000; 86: 782–9.

54. Uzzo RG, Wei JT, Hafez K et al. Comparison of direct hospital cost and length of stay for radical nephrectomy versus nephron-sparing surgery in the management of localized renal cell carcinoma. Urol 1999; 54: 994–8.

55. Schvarts O, Tsui Ke-Hung, Smith RB et al. Blood loss and the need for transfusion in patients who undergo partial or radical nephrectomy for renal cell carcinoma. J Urol 2000; 164: 1160–3.

56. Drachenberg DE, Mena OJ, Choyke PL et al. Parenchymal sparing surgery for central renal tumors in patients with hereditary renal cancers. J Urol 2004; 172: 49–53.

57. Hafez KS, Fergany AF, Novick AC. Nephron sparing surgery for localized renal cell carcinoma: impact of tumor size on patient survival, tumor recurrence, and TNM staging. J Urol 1999; 162: 1930–3.

58. Fergany AF, Hafez KS, Novick AC. Long-term results of nephron sparing surgery for localized renal cell carcinoma: 10-year follow up. J Urol 2000; 163: 442–5.

59. D'Armiento M, Damiano R, Feleppa B et al. Elective conservative surgery for renal carcinoma versus radical nephrectomy: a prospective study. BJU Int 1997; 79: 15–19.

60. Lau WKO, Blute ML, Weaver A et al. Matched comparison of radical nephrectomy vs nephron-sparing surgery in patients with unilateral renal cell carcinoma and a normal contralateral kidney. Mayo Clin Proc 2000; 75: 1236–42.

7

Minimally invasive approaches for renal cell carcinoma: an overview

Marshall S Wingo and Raymond J Leveillee

INTRODUCTION

Widespread use of abdominal imaging has increased the number of incidental tumors found in the greater than 38 000 renal masses diagnosed in the United States in 2006.[1] Thirteen percent of all renal tumors were discovered incidentally in the 1980s. By the mid 1990s incidental lesions accounted for 60% of all renal masses.[2] These incidental lesions present at a lower stage, grade, and likelihood of metastasis, and have improved survival outcomes compared to tumors detected in symptomatic patients.[2–4] A significant number of these lesions will ultimately prove benign, but this diagnosis is difficult to obtain preoperatively. Imaging techniques are unable to consistently predict pathology and percutaneous renal biopsy is unreliable with an accuracy of only 76 to 80%.[5]

The potential 'overtreatment' of incidental small renal lesions with radical nephrectomy, along with a desire to reduce patient morbidity and preserve renal function, led to the development of nephron-sparing techniques and minimally invasive methods to manage renal tumors. Nephron-sparing surgery (NSS) was initially indicated for patients with localized renal cell carcinoma (RCC) combined with a compromised contralateral kidney and a need to preserve overall renal function, but now has become applicable in patients with a single, unilateral, localized RCC with a normal contralateral renal unit.[6]

Nephron-sparing surgery began with the partial nephrectomy (PN). The technique has evolved and for tumors less than 4 cm in diameter PN has the same oncologic efficacy as radical nephrectomy as defined by local tumor recurrence rates.[7,8] Open PN remains the standard for NSS, but extensive experience with laparoscopic PN at many centers has made the procedures virtually equivalent in oncologic outcome, although higher complication rates have been demonstrated when compared to open PN.[9] Laparoscopic approaches are typically indicated in smaller, more peripherally located tumors and offer the advantages of reduced postoperative narcotic usage, shorter hospital stays, and faster return to normal activity level compared to open surgery. Although laparoscopic PN can reduce patient convalescence, it can be technically demanding. Large volume blood loss, transfusions, urinary leak, and functional loss from prolonged warm ischemia during intraoperative occlusion of the hilar vessels has been described. Complication rates have declined with the evolution of the laparoscopic PN technique and accumulated surgeon experience, but the operation continues to require proficiency in advanced laparoscopic skills.

An improved understanding in the biology of RCC and the impact of laparoscopic PN in the treatment of small renal tumors encouraged clinicians to search for more widely available, less invasive means of treating renal masses. Renal ablative techniques were developed to offer widespread application and improved patient procedural morbidity, and to reduce the potential for complications. A large variety of generators, ablation probes, and energy delivery systems are now commercially available.

PATIENT SELECTION

As NSS became more widely accepted ablative therapies were developed as an alternative for elderly patients, patients with multiple tumors such as those with von Hippel–Lindau disease, those with compromised renal function, and patients with comorbid conditions who were felt to be inappropriate candidates for surgical resection. Faced with an increasingly older population, often with multiple medical comorbidities and a growing incidence of small renal masses, the ability to offer a minimally invasive ablative therapy was theoretically advantageous. As clinical experience has accumulated, ablative therapies are now offered for many small to medium sized tumors, despite unavailable long-term clinical efficacy data.

Energy-based tissue ablative techniques include radiofrequency ablation (RFA), cryoablation, high-intensity focused ultrasound (HIFU), microwave therapy, and interstitial photon irradiation. Originally renal tumor ablations were performed through open incisions, but now can be applied through laparoscopic or more commonly percutaneous routes.

The primary requirement for an ablative technology to be efficacious is that it must deliver a lethal treatment to the cancer cells, leaving no viable cancer cells within the treated area. Of equal importance, the surgeon must be able to localize, control, and predict the area of treatment, while avoiding the inadvertent ablation of surrounding healthy tissue. Ablative therapies, when applied correctly in appropriately selected patients, can achieve these treatment goals.

RADIOFREQUENCY ABLATION

Indications for radiofrequency ablation treatment

RFA is a heat-based means of tissue destruction originally developed for the treatment of aberrant cardiac pathways. The first oncologic application involved the treatment of primary and metastatic liver tumors.[10,11] Current applications include the treatment of breast malignancy, aberrant cardiac pathways, gynecologic tumors, prostate disease, bone lesions, pancreatic cancer, renal tumors,[12] and metastatic lesions. Zagoria et al[13] successfully treated two small lung nodules as the sole manifestation of metastatic disease. Gervais et al reported successful treatment of lymph node metastases with RFA from ovarian, prostate, and renal primary tumors.[14]

With reports of RFA success in renal tumors ranging from small incidental lesions to metastatic deposits, how do we determine who is appropriate for renal RFA treatment? Prospective randomized clinical series to identify patients appropriate for RFA therapy have not been performed to date. Phase II trials have included patients receiving RFA simultaneously with open or laparoscopic nephrectomy, prior to nephrectomy, patients deemed inappropriate for extirpative surgery due to comorbidities, and patients with hereditary RCC. Most clinicians agree that patients with a solitary kidney,

multiple synchronous RCC, von Hippel–Lindau disease, familial RCC, or limited renal function are appropriate candidates for RFA treatment, but controversy exists in younger patients without significant comorbid conditions, normal contralateral renal function, and minimal future risk of renal function loss. McAchran et al selects patients with small, peripherally-oriented tumors (<4 cm) who are not surgical candidates and have a life expectancy of greater than 4 months as appropriate for RFA treatment. However, patients with small renal lesions who specifically request RFA therapy are also considered.[15] As experience with RFA accumulates, intermediate and long-term results will become available. Favorable outcomes will justify the treatment of smaller, potentially less-aggressive tumors in younger, healthier patients with RFA therapy.

Technologic background

Radiofrequency energy is composed of an alternating electrical current (AC) with a wavelength between 10 kHz and 900 MHz. Commercially available RF generators typically produce current at frequencies from 400 to 500 kHz.[16] Energy is traditionally delivered through a monopolar circuit. Current emanates from the RF generator through the electrode, passes through the patient's tissues, and returns to the generator through a grounding pad on the skin. Impedance (ohms, Ω) or resistance to flow of current exists within the circuit and varies according to the tissue density and composition. RF energy delivered through a bipolar circuit begins at the electrode and returns through an additional electrode in close proximity to the point of origin. This circuit type minimizes the amount of tissue traversed by the electrical current and offers certain advantages and disadvantages to be discussed.

Body tissues responsive to electrical energy such as nerve and muscle tissue can be stimulated at frequencies under 1000 Hz, but not by frequencies of 10 kHz or greater. The discovery of this principle fostered the use of electrical energy in surgery, beginning with Edwin Beer in 1910 during transurethral resection of bladder tumors. Work continued with Henry Bugbee (1913) and his electrode to treat bladder neck obstruction, Max Stern (1926) with resectotherm of the prostate, and William Bovie and Harvey Cushing (1928) who laid the groundwork for modern electrosurgery.[17,18]

To fully understand radiofrequency ablative therapies a few electrical terms must be defined. An RF current, measured in amperes (A) is defined as a flow of electrons from the orbit of one atom to the orbit of another. The current flows through a closed circuit from a cathode to an anode and always follows a path of least electrical resistance. Impedance to current flow is described as the resistance to the flow of electrons in an alternating-current circuit, measured in ohms. The effects of radiofrequency tissue ablation are mediated through the transfer of heat. As the current is propagated from the generator, through the probe, into the tissues, and returns to the generator, impedance to the flow of current naturally exists in the tissues. The component of current that cannot freely continue its flow in the circuit disperses into the tissue, resulting in molecular agitation. The molecular agitation releases energy locally and is transformed into heat. It is this heat 'byproduct' that causes the tissue injury.

The mathematical properties of RFA are described by the bio-heat equation developed by Pennes:[19]

$$\frac{\rho c \partial T}{\partial t} = \Delta k \Delta T + m_b c_b (T_a - T) + q_v$$

Where ρ is tissue density in kg/m^3; c is the tissue-specific heat at constant pressure in $J/kg°C$; c_b is the blood-specific heat at constant pressure in $J/kg°C$; k is the thermal conductivity of the tissue in $W/m°C$; m_b is the the blood perfusion rate at a specific arterial size in kg/sm^3; q_v is the volumetric heat generation rate in W/m^3; t is time in seconds; T is transient tissue temperature in °C; and T_a is arterial temperature at a specific arterial size in °C.

The left-hand term is the specific absorption rate (SAR) and describes the change in temperature of the tissue over time. This value is derived from the sum of three terms. $\Delta k \Delta T$ describes the conductive heat loss in the tissue, $m_b c_b (T_a - T)$ describes the capacitive heat loss in the tissue, and the term q_v represents the contribution of heat from any externally applied power source such as an RF generator.

All variables are measurable within a specific tissue type, allowing an accurate prediction of the RF lesion size and extent given the applied intensity and duration of the generated current. Since these thermal properties can vary with different tissue types and tissue characteristics, using an identical generator, probe, and current setting may result in a range of RF lesion sizes in different organ systems.

As seen in the above equation, a temperature equilibrium is reached at a given level of applied current. As the distance away from the probe tip increases, the loss of capacitive and conductive heat from the tissue is equal to the heat applied from the external energy source. After this steady state is reached, with additional time the RF lesion does not increase in size. Longer ablation cycles do not result in larger RF lesions, only longer temperature exposure for the specific lesion size.

The importance of impedance

As electrical current flows through a circuit, an impediment to flow may occur. Electrical current flow is analogous to the flow of water through a garden hose. If one puts a finger over the open end of the hose or kinks the tubing, pressure and heat within the tubing increase. Similarly, the natural resistance to the flow of current that occurs in the tissues, manifested as increased impedance, generates heat and subsequent tissue damage. If the impedance rises too rapidly (i.e., the current density is too high) heating occurs too rapidly and tissue desiccation will ensue. If the impedance near the electrode is high, an elevated current density will result in desiccation, carbonization, and eschar formation in the adjacent tissue, insulating the probe and further preventing the spread of energy to the surrounding tissues.[16] Tissue heating will be limited to a small localized area surrounding the probe and cannot reach the outer margins of the renal malignancy. Impedance must be controlled for effective RF treatment.

Plain or 'dry' electrodes

The first RF experiments were performed with plain metal electrodes. Plain electrode RFA involves the delivery of current through a single, expandable, or bipolar electrode without the assistance of cooling or 'wet' techniques. Conventional plain RF electrodes are limited in tissue ablation efficiency by high current densities at the metal electrode–tissue interface. High current densities result in high temperatures (>100°C) followed by tissue desiccation and charring very close to the electrode surface (<1 mm). The resultant charring raises the impedance of the tissue and prevents the propagation of current to tissues further from the electrode.[20]

To improve the propagation of RF energy and reduce the restriction of high electrode–tissue interface impedance, investigators have tried to manipulate several variables in the RF circuit. Engineers have limited the maximum voltage applied through the electrode to prevent arcing, developed a negative feedback circuit limiting the applied power when the impedance rises, and installed a thermal sensor at the electrode tip to maintain the temperature below 100°C by reducing the power applied to the circuit (VidaMed, Freemont, CA; RITA-Medical Systems, Mountain View, CA; Medtronic, Minneapolis, MN). These maneuvers have resulted in mixed success. Attempts to reduce the electrode temperature and tissue impedance through reduction of the power applied to the circuit limit the amount, rate, and total volume of tissue treated. Theoretic limits in RF lesion size exist in plain electrode systems.

Investigators realized that applying a level of current appropriate to treat larger renal lesions required an ability to manipulate the impedance to current flow within the surrounding tissues. Strategies to manipulate the tissue–electrode interface impedance resulted in the development of alternate RF probe configurations. Single-shaft RF electrodes include plain, cooled, expandable, bipolar, and wet configurations. Multiple electrode systems are also available and classified according to probe number, electric mode, activation mode, and electrode type (i.e., plain, wet, cooled, expandable).[21]

Cell destruction by the application of thermal energy

RF ablative techniques convert radiant energy into thermal energy in the tissues, ultimately leading to coagulative necrosis. Damage is believed to manifest through protein denaturation, DNA/RNA chain disruption, and to some degree vascular congestion. Effective ablation and cell damage is a time–temperature-dependent process. Both lower heat and higher heat damage tissue and result in cell death equivalently, but more time is required at lower temperatures. It may require hours to achieve cell kill at a temperature of 45°C, but will instantaneously occur at a temperature of 100°C. High temperatures result in immediately identifiable cellular changes including obvious structural damage, desiccation, vaporization, and carbonization. Lower temperatures are associated with less grossly apparent changes including denatured cellular enzymes, damaged membrane channels, and after several hours cellular edema, organelle swelling, and blebing. Elevated temperatures cause the intracellular buffering capacity and transport mechanisms to fail, causing an overload of intracellular calcium and cell death. Disruption of the delicate intracellular balance causes localized inflammatory changes to appear followed by an ischemic response leading to acidosis and eventual coagulative necrosis.

Following thermal injury the basic structure of the cell is preserved. Between 3 and 7 days after RF treatment the damaged tissue begins to show signs of coagulative necrosis with interspersed inflammatory cells. The necrotic debris is then removed by fragmentation or phagocytosis. Concomitant apoptosis can increase the total area of cell kill through the promotion of nuclear pyknosis in cells adjacent to directly injured cells.[16] All evidence of organized renal cellular architecture disappears by 30 days. The necrotic tissue absorbed with fragmentation and phagocytosis transforms into avascular scar tissue that may become smaller in size and does not enhance on contrasted imaging.[22,23]

In experimental models, tissue ablation occurs when the temperature is elevated for a sufficient period of time as determined by the tissue specific time–temperature curve for necrosis.[24] Tissue destruction has been previously shown to occur at a temperature of approximately 50°C when maintained for 15 seconds or 55°C reported in the literature.[25–27] At temperatures between 60 and 100°C irreversible damage occurs almost instantaneously. At this temperature the damage to mitochondria and cytosolic enzymes is immediate and unrecoverable. Experimental models based on thermal treatment of malignant tissue have shown cell death in tissue exposed for 1 hour at 43°C. Each elevation of 1°C reduces the time necessary for cell kill by half.

Extrapolating these time–temperature data supports the idea of instantaneous cell kill at a temperature of 50°C (Figure 7.1).

'Heat-sink' considerations

Tissue vascularity within and surrounding the renal tumor may affect the volume of the ablated area. Adjacent blood flow may dissipate the generated heat, resulting in a 'heat-sink' phenomenon, making it more challenging to treat highly vascular lesions and lesions adjacent to larger blood vessels such as the renal hilum. Attempts have been made by researchers to reduce this effect by clamping the renal hilum during treatment. Corwin et al utilized clamping of the renal hilum in a swine model and demonstrated that the ablated lesion size was larger in the ischemic kidneys than in the normally perfused cohort. However, when researchers examined the kidneys 1 month after treatment, no difference in lesion size was detectable.[28] Chang et al examined a swine model using renal arterial embolization and hilar clamping as preferred occlusion methods and found

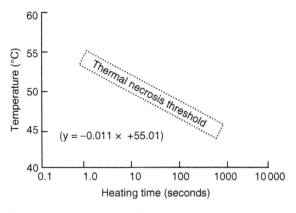

Figure 7.1 Temperature–time relationship.

lesions to be of similar size between the ischemic techniques and twice the volume of the lesions in the nonischemic kidneys.[29] Although clamping of the renal hilum is not possible in percutaneous procedures, research examining selective arterial constriction and embolization of renal tumor vasculature prior to RF ablation is ongoing.

Electrode overview

Modern imaging techniques can accurately characterize most renal masses. Clinicians using axial, sagittal, coronal, and in many cases three-dimensional rendering not only know the size and shape of the lesion, but can also determine with great accuracy the vascular supply, cystic vs solid component, and proximity of adjacent structures. The goal of therapy should be the creation of a zone of heat that includes the entire volume of the mass and extends an extra 1–5 mm beyond the tumor edge to achieve an acceptable treatment margin.

Predicting the size of the 'zone of kill'

The volume, shape, and lethal potential of RF is dependent on several interacting variables. Applied current can vary in intensity, duration, and pattern. Tissue properties including impedance, density, hydration status, vascular supply, and susceptibility to thermal injury can be very different. Ablation electrodes are constructed with variety in their needle number, pattern, and deployment depth as well as cooling mechanisms and temperature monitoring ability. All factors interact to determine the success or failure of the ablation technique.

Treatment of renal tumors with RF energy begins by selecting a circuit type. There are two ways to deliver electrical energy to the tissue and specific electrodes associated with each type. With monopolar radiofrequency ablation the patient becomes an integral part of the circuit as electrons flow from the electrode, through the patient's tissues, and exit at the ground or return plate. A large grounding pad is used in order to disperse the returning current over a large surface area, reducing the current density at the skin–grounding pad interface. In monopolar circuits, the majority of the current density is focused around the probe tip. Lesion size is determined by the ability of the current to propagate in all directions, radially into the surrounding tissues.

Unfortunately, accidental burns are a potential complication of monopolar therapy. The current always seeks the path of least resistance. If the grounding pad faults, the electrons will exit the body at an alternate site to complete the circuit. If current exits the body at a site other than the grounding pad it must overcome the impedance of the skin, requiring a build-up of charge and typically resulting in a skin burn.

As an alternative, bipolar RF involves an isolated circuit with current flowing from an active electrode and returning within a receiving electrode located either on the same needle or between adjacent needles (Figure 7.2). The majority of the ablated tissue lies along the current path between the electrodes, allowing for a predictable ablation volume. In a bipolar system current flows through the tissue for a limited distance, exiting at the path of least resistance, the return electrode. Due to the closed loop circuit with limited tissue exposure, these systems reduce the hazards of stray current and electrical complications, but may have limitations in RF lesion geometry and size.

Most renal tumors are either spherical or conical in shape. On radiographic imaging they are often described utilizing two or three dimensions and an estimated volume is calculated. For simplicity we describe the volume of a sphere in mathematical terms as:

$$V = \frac{4}{3}\pi r^3$$

where V = volume and r = radius. As the radius increases, the volume of the sphere (tumor) increases dramatically. For example; a 2 cm diameter tumor ($r = 1.0$ cm) has a volume = $4 \times 1 \times 1 \times 1 = 4$ cc. If the radius doubles to 2 cm, then the volume is now $4 \times 2 \times 2 \times 2 = 32$ cc! Ablation of small tumors can be readily achieved because the spread of heat is less influenced by local characteristics such as fat content and blood flow. As the required ablation volume increases it becomes more challenging to insure uniformity and adequacy.

Electrical current flowing through tissues creates heat as a byproduct of molecular agitation caused by the tissue impedance. In a self-limiting way, if the current density increases the tissue becomes overheated, sometimes to the point of vaporization or carbonization, and the ablation volume reaches a theoretic limit. In order to overcome limitations in RF lesion size

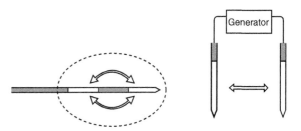

Figure 7.2 Bipolar RF circuit.

investigators have attempted to decrease the current density to allow for wider delivery of higher amounts of current.

One strategy involves increasing the electrode size, a situation undesirable from a minimally invasive perspective. Alternatively, current may be applied at low levels to prevent overheating, but this strategy leads to exceedingly long treatment times. Other approaches to reduce the current density include using cluster or expandable probes, electrodes that alter the local environment by infusing the area surrounding the probe with a conducting fluid, or internally cooled electrodes. In the next section, we discuss the various electrodes available and the ablation characteristics of each.

Electrode systems

Mulier et al proposed a standardized nomenclature for RF electrode systems. Single-shaft RF electrodes are described as plain, cooled, expandable, bipolar, or wet. Cooled electrodes are further classified as single or clustered. Expandable electrodes include the subcategories multitined and coiled. Some of these features can occur simultaneously along a single-shaft electrode and are referred to as double and triple combination designs. Multiple electrode systems are classified by the number of probes, circuit type (monopolar or bipolar), activation mode (consecutive, simultaneous, or switching), site of insertion, and the electrode system (wet, cooled, or expandable).[21] A standardized nomenclature system allows more accurate comparison of technologies and a better understanding of published RF techniques.

Single-shaft RF electrodes

Small renal tumors may be adequately treated with a single-shaft electrode depending on probe characteristics and the ability to propagate lethal temperatures to the tumor periphery. Generally, lesions less than 2–3 cm in diameter may be treated with a single-shaft ablation probe system. Plain RF electrode characteristics and limitations have been discussed previously. Improvements in single-shaft electrode systems have been developed. The most commonly utilized single-shaft electrodes and their characteristics are now described.

Wet RF electrodes
In RF applications, the energy applied to the surrounding tissue is described by the equation:

$$q_a = \frac{|J|^2}{\sigma}$$

where J is the current density in amps/m^2 and σ is the electrical conductivity of the tissue in σ/m. As seen from the equation, an increase in the electrical conductivity of the tissue would result in less power and heat within the tissue adjacent to the electrode. Heat would be propagated further down the circuit and closer to the grounding pad. Haines and Watson were able to demonstrate during RFA of canine right ventricular wall myocardium that an increasingly concentrated saline infusion applied adjacent to the RF electrode reduced the current density at the electrode–tissue interface and allowed the resultant heat to propagate further from the electrode into the surrounding myocardial tissue. Investigators discovered that the saline was such an effective conductor of current that temperatures were actually higher away from the electrode than at the tissue–electrode interface.[30]

Thus 'wet' RFA was developed in an attempt to avoid the problem of high tissue temperatures at the electrode–tissue interface (Figure 7.3) In these original systems, interstitial saline was infused during the simultaneous application of RF energy. Saline spreads the current density and heat away from the electrode and out into the tissue, creating a larger ablation zone. Hoey et al compared dry RFA with wet RFA utilizing 14% NaCl and 37% NaCl in a canine liver model.[31] After 10 W had been applied for 30 seconds the tissue adjacent to the dry electrode rose above 150°C, but the tissue 2–6 mm away did not rise above 50°C. With the infusion of 37% NaCl the temperature 6 mm from the electrode was equal to the tissue temperature immediately adjacent to the electrode (Figure 7.4). Heat had been effectively propagated without desiccating the tissues. These results suggested that a larger, more reproducible lesion could be produced with the wet probe. Leveillee and Hoey et al further compared conventional RF and RF with saline perfusion (14.6% NaCl) in a dog prostate model and demonstrated that saline pretreatment created larger lesions (mean 8.5 cm) than conventional RF (mean 0.34 cm).[31]

Cooled electrodes
As an alternative to control the current density and high temperatures at the electrode–tissue interface probes were

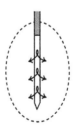
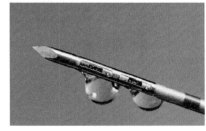

Figure 7.3 Wet electrode.

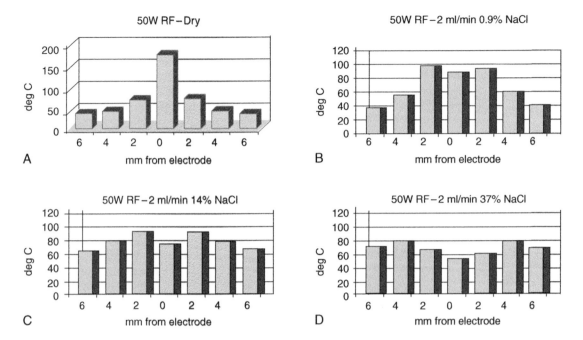

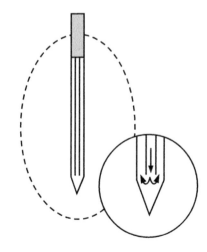

Figure 7.4 Radiofrequency ablation of canine liver. From Hoey et al.[31] (A) Dry electrode, (B) 0.9% NaCl, (C) 14% NaCl, (D) 37% NaCl.

designed to be internally cooled. In the Cool-Tip™ system (Valleylab, Boulder, CO) water is continuously circulated through the electrode in an impedance controlled system (Figure 7.5). Cooled water circulated through the electrode tip prevents tissue immediately adjacent to the probe from reaching >100°C.[32] This technology prevents tissue desiccation and allows the current to propagate further into the tissues, creating a larger treatment field.

Initial experience with this type of electrode came from Gervais et al, who were able to ablate tumors as large as 5.0 cm.[33] Pereira et al compared perfused electrodes, cooled-tip, 9-tine, and 12-tine electrodes in pig livers and found that larger lesions were created with the perfused and cooled-tip electrodes. They found that the multitined devices resulted in a spherical lesion and were more consistent in the ablated volume.[34] Walther et al[35] at the National Cancer Institute have reported using a cooled-tip system since 2001 in conjunction with a 200 W generator. They percutaneously and laparoscopically ablated 8 and 12 hereditary type tumors, respectively. At a median follow-up of over 1 year, no recurrence has been identified by contrast enhancement on CT imaging.

Figure 7.5 Cooled electrode.

Multitined expandable electrodes

Multiple tined electrodes have been developed for RFA application (Figure 7.6). They increase the overall ablation volume while maintaining a lower current density at each individual tine–tissue interface. The use of multiple tines, in an umbrella or 'Christmas tree' configuration, greatly increases the ablation area. Current is transmitted through the individual tines with each effectively acting as a separate needle ablation probe. RF lesions appear around each tine as a sphere or elliptical shaped area of coagulative necrosis that

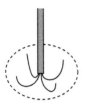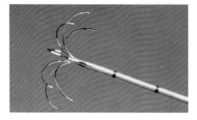

Figure 7.6 Multitined expandable electrode (RITA-Medical Systems, Mountain View, CA).

envelops the electrode. The tines are positioned within the tumor so that the ablation fields overlap to cover the entire tumor volume without skipped areas of treatment. Tumors of up to 7 cm in size have been ablated with these probe configurations utilizing overlapping ablation fields.[36,37]

Bipolar electrodes

RFA using bipolar probes eliminates the need for a grounding pad. Energy is delivered from the generator, through the cathode, and returns through the anode positioned in close proximity on the same probe array (Figure 7.2). Tissue destruction occurs with the tissue between the two probes and is generally of a uniform geometry, but can in some cases extend beyond the needles.[38] Nakada et al compared monopolar and bipolar lesions created in in-vivo and ex-vivo porcine kidneys. A 1.5 cm lesion was produced with a conventional dry monopolar electrode while a bipolar electrode with a 3 cm separation between cathode and anode produced a 2.8 cm diameter lesion on average.[39] The authors concluded that larger lesions were possible with a bipolar arrangement.

Multiple electrode systems

Multiple electrode systems are composed of multiple single-shaft electrodes, utilized together in order to ablate larger renal lesions effectively.

Single 'dry' needle electrodes have limitations with respect to the volume of ablation that they can achieve. Creation of larger lesions could be achieved by increasing the surface area (i.e., the diameter) of the probe, but this becomes impractical when trying to minimize tissue trauma and reduce invasiveness. Propagation of current to the outer periphery of large tumors requires a large amplitude current, maintenance of a low current density at the electrode–tissue interface, and favorable tissue impedance. Current and current density are not mutually exclusive, therefore treating a large tumor

with an energy level necessary for tumor destruction is limited by the density and resultant heat generated. Effective temperatures for cell kill 1–5 mm beyond the periphery of a large tumor may be theoretically impossible with a single 'dry' system electrode or even with 'wet' and internally cooled single probes due to current density restraints. Multiple electrode configurations were developed to treat these larger lesions. Multiple electrode systems are classified by the number of probes, circuit type (monopolar or bipolar), activation mode (consecutive, simultaneous, or switching), site of insertion, and the electrode system (wet, cooled, or expandable).[21] These systems offer the same advantages and disadvantages as the single probe technologies they are built from.

Multiple single-shaft electrode systems

An alternative approach to treating larger renal tumors involves the placement of multiple single needle electrodes into the tumor separated by small distances. This process subdivides the tumor, with each area of the mass treated individually in overlapping segments. Monopolar and bipolar configurations are used, with current passing from electrode to adjacent electrode in the bipolar circuits (Figure 7.7). Current is activated either consecutively (the second electrode is activated after the first), simultaneously, or in a rapid switching mode. Switch-box systems are available for multiple electrodes that automatically rotate the applied current from electrode to electrode (Figure 7.8). A larger volume of ablation is achieved by taking advantage of the pulsing phenomenon of current allowing the temperature at each electrode to be lower overall and the current to propagate further.[40] In very large tumors the needle set can be repositioned and the lesion retreated with a different ablation configuration.

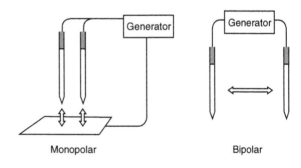

Figure 7.7 Monopolar and bipolar multiple single-shaft electrode systems.

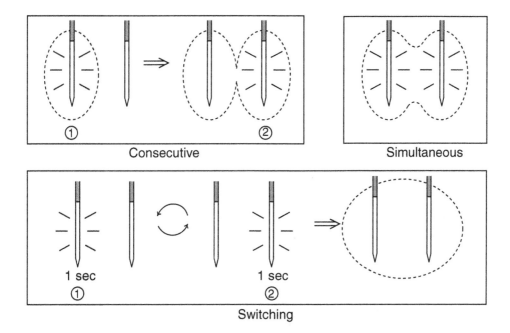

Figure 7.8 Multiple single-shaft electrode systems activation modes.

Overview of radiofrequency ablation technique

Patient selection

RF treatment may be performed through either a percutaneous or laparoscopic approach. Preoperative imaging is helpful in choosing the appropriate modality. Anteriorly or laterally oriented tumors commonly involve bowel segments that obstruct direct anterior percutaneous access to the renal lesion and may rest in close proximity to the anticipated thermal field. In these cases laparoscopic mobilization of the bowel, exposure of the tumor surface, and directly visualized insertion of the ablation probe into the tumor parenchyma is indicated for both efficacy and safety (Figure 7.9). Laparoscopic exposure reduces the risk of thermal injury to adjacent organs. In addition to intestinal mobilization and protection, laparoscopic approaches allow separation of other vital structures including the ureter and renal pelvis from the ablation zone (Figure 7.10). The authors have not experienced thermal damage to the ureter, renal pelvis, vasculature, or bowel when diligent dissection and mobilization were performed.

Purely percutaneous RF treatment with the assistance of radiologic imaging may be performed in posteriorly oriented tumors (Figure 7.11). Direct percutaneous needle access to the lesion may be obtained with particular

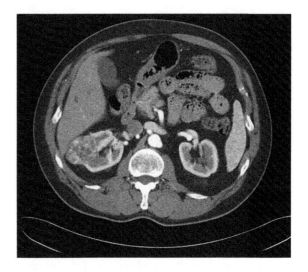

Figure 7.9 Laterally oriented renal tumor for laparoscopic-assisted RFA.

attention paid to avoiding injury to the pleural cavity, lung parenchyma, or posteriorly oriented bowel segments. The avoidance of laparoscopic abdominal manipulation, insufflation, and mobilization raises the possibility of RF treatment performed as an outpatient procedure with a shorter period of convalescence.

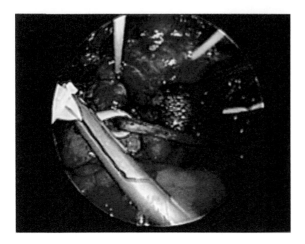

Figure 7.10

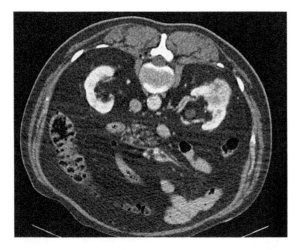

Figure 7.11 Posteriorly oriented renal tumor for CT-guided RFA (prone position).

Monitoring treatment area and ablated lesion size

You cannot see heat. Precise placement of the ablation probe within the lesion and subsequent monitoring of the treatment area are the central challenges of RFA therapy. The probe tip and ablation area cannot be directly visualized, therefore radiographic imaging modalities are essential during the treatment process. In peripheral temperature-monitoring cases, ultrasound, CT, or MRI is used initially to place temperature probes in the correct location and depth at the tumor periphery (Figure 7.12). CT and MRI can then be used to assess ablated area volume and enhancement after each treatment cycle. Determining the size of the radiofrequency lesion in real

time is difficult, because most tissue changes are not immediately visible. Damage to the tumor vasculature tends to be readily apparent during and after ablation, with changes in enhancement pattern predictive of treatment completeness. Residual enhancement can be targeted with a radiographically directed retreatment cycle.

Ultrasound, CT, and MRI have been investigated in RFA therapy. Ultrasound monitoring is helpful to position the ablation probe and peripheral temperature probes prior to treatment, but becomes limited during ablation by electrical interference from the radiofrequency probe as well as microbubble formation at the lesion periphery that limits visualization. Animal studies suggest that contrast-medium enhancement combined with ultrasound may allow real-time assessment of the ablation process.[41] Cadeddu et al examined lesions created with porcine kidneys with contrast-enhanced ultrasonography and found that ultrasound accurately predicted the lesion size and geometry, concluding that ultrasound appeared to be an accurate method to monitor RFA treatment.[42,43] This method, however, has not gained widespread acceptance.

Su et al[44] accumulated experience using CT fluoroscopy for percutaneous needle guidance in 37 treatments. Images provided excellent visualization of the needle entering the tumor, allowed investigators to avoid adjacent organs, and were able to determine the degree of vascular enhancement postablation. CT scans performed postoperatively characteristically reveal a diminished level of contrast enhancement, but an increase in fat stranding, and soft tissue edema in completely treated renal lesions. Although contrast can pool in the vasculature due to thermally-induced inflammation surrounding the tumor, most successful treatments are non-enhancing.

Postoperative MRI has been shown by investigators to differentiate between untreated and treated tissue to within 2 mm of accuracy when confirmed by pathologic results.[45] Lewin et al extended the use of MRI to real-time ablation monitoring in phase II trials. MRI was used to perform percutaneous renal RFA and the resultant lesions were observed as enlarging low-intensity lesions surrounded by higher-intensity tissue on T2-weighting. Investigators utilized these enhancement characteristics to reposition probes for subsequent RF cycles if the high-intensity T2 signal persisted.[46] MRI was used to target renal lesions in 10 patients with no recurrences detected at a mean of 25 months' follow-up. Advantages to MRI include excellent soft tissue and vascular visualization, high resolution, flexibility in image reconstruction, and the future potential for temperature sensing.

Peripheral fiber-optic temperature monitoring has been developed as a means to perform real-time monitoring during the RFA treatment. Using a combination of direct visualization and CT or ultrasound guidance,

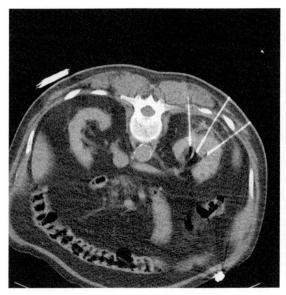
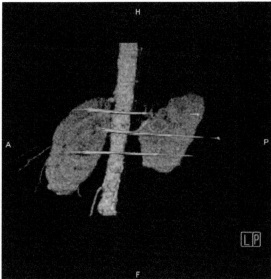

Figure 7.12 CT-guided placement of peripheral temperature-sensing probes.

non-conducting fiber-optic temperature probes are inserted into the tumor periphery and positioned 5 mm from the tumor–parenchymal interface at the superior, inferior, lateral, and medial margins (Lumasense, Santa Clara, CA). Continuous temperature measurements are returned from each probe during the ablation. RFA continues until all peripheral temperatures exceed the predetermined level and duration. RFA probes can be repositioned and a treatment cycle performed if a region of the tumor periphery does not reach the desired temperature. The authors' experience with this technique in over 135 tumors treated has resulted in two tumors requiring RFA retreatment and only one lesion with persistent radiographic enhancement identified with residual pathologically confirmed malignancy.[47]

Peripheral temperature monitoring has the additional benefit of helping to protect vital structures during RFA treatment. Fibers can be positioned between the renal pelvis, vasculature, or ureter and the renal mass to ensure temperatures do not exceed the tolerances of these structures.

Generator and treatment control types

Radiofrequency energy can be applied at a wide variety of current intensities and lengths of time. Undertreatment with low intensity or shorter intervals and overtreatment with tissue desiccation due to high-intensity and prolonged cycles are equally ineffective. Currently available RFA systems tailor the delivery of current through feedback systems based on either temperature or impedance.

Temperature based systems

Temperature-based systems work by monitoring the temperature at the electrode tip and adjusting the energy delivered to maintain a specific temperature for a specific treatment duration. As the impedance at the electrode–tissue interface increases, the temperature at the electrode tip will rise. The generator reduces the current to avoid tissue desiccation and charring. An inherent limitation in this control system is that the temperature elsewhere within the tumor may not match the temperature recorded at the electrode tip. Without peripheral temperature recording, this method introduces an uncertainty in the adequacy of the treatment at the tumor periphery. To achieve an effective temperature at the tumor periphery a higher temperature must be tolerated at the probe tip with a decline in temperature level assumed as the distance from the probe center increases.

Impedance-based systems

Impedance-controlled systems measure the tissue impedance at the electrode–tissue interface. Radiofrequency energy is delivered until the impedance rises above a maximum allowed increase (i.e., 20 ohms). When the tissue impedance exceeds this level tissues become desiccated, carbonization occurs, and the tissue is no longer viable. The tissue adjacent to the electrode now acts as an insulator, preventing further propagation of the energy into the tumor periphery. A limitation in this control system is that no temperature or impedance information is available for tissues beyond the surface of the electrode. Although during current delivery the impedance level may not exceed established limits, temperatures at the renal tumor periphery may not reach levels sufficient for tissue destruction. Tissue impedances vary with tissue type, water content, fat composition, and cellular architecture.

Both systems are thought to provide equivalent renal ablation efficacy in animal models.[48] However, Rehman et al found temperature-based RFA to provide a more uniform necrosis pattern when compared to impedance control. He noted that the impedance-based system caused skip lesions which contained viable cells.[49] Both methods fail to deliver information about temperatures and the tumor periphery. Temperature- and impedance-based systems prevent desiccation and carbonization at the electrode–tissue interface, but do not guarantee lethal temperatures throughout the lesion. Peripheral temperature-monitoring techniques or temperature-capable imaging modalities help to add confidence that treatments are adequate.

CT-guided RF treatment

CT-guided RFA can be performed under general anesthesia, intravenous sedation, or after infiltration of a local anesthetic. It is done with the cooperative efforts of the interventional radiologist and the urologist. The patient is placed in a prone or full-flank position to provide percutaneous access to the retroperitoneum. After preoperative imaging is reviewed by the team, probe type, location, and circuit type are determined based on tumor characteristics, size, and anatomic relation to other structures. If peripheral temperature monitoring is performed, a minimum of three fiberoptic temperature sensors (LumaSense, Santa Clara, CA) are placed under CT guidance at the peripheral (superior, inferior, lateral, medial) and deep margins of the tumor, 5 mm from the tumor–parenchymal interface. The probes are inserted through non-conducting sheaths of standard 18 gauge needles (TLA or Yueh), found in a typical interventional radiology suite.

Biopsies of the tumor are obtained with a spring-loaded (i.e., Tru-Cut) biopsy needle prior to the RF ablation cycle.

The RF probe(s) is positioned under CT guidance, percutaneously between the previously placed temperature probes, directed toward the center of the tumor and advanced until the deep margin is reached with the probe tip.

After the temperature sensors and ablation needle are properly positioned the RF cycle is initiated.

The ablation is complete after a specified time interval, when the target temperature or impedance is reached at the probe tip or, in the case of peripheral temperature monitoring, when all the target temperatures have been achieved. In our practice the cycle is monitored and performed under the guidance of the surgeon urologist. Manipulation and alternate targeting of the RF probe and repeat application of RF energy may be necessary to achieve the target temperature at all monitored sites.

A CT-guided approach is appropriate for posteriorly-oriented tumors. Particular attention is paid to the large intestine and pleural cavity. Avoidance of a low lying posterior pleural cavity may be achieved through an angled, oblique percutaneous approach, but alternative approaches should be considered if pleural violation is inevitable. Several methods of bowel manipulation have been described. Saline solution or CO_2 injection has been used with RFA to increase separation between vital structures and the renal lesion.

Rendon et al, using a porcine model, developed a method of hydro and gas dissection to protect the bowel from thermal injury. Saline or CO_2 was injected through a percutaneously placed needle between the renal capsule and Gerota's fascia, creating a thermal cushion layer.[50] No adverse effects were noted. Farrell et al applied the technique of hydrodissection with sterile water to protect the bowel during a human RFA case.[51] Yamakado et al described the placement of balloon catheters to displace the duodenum and stomach adjacent to liver tumors during RF therapy.[52] Margulis et al described a technique of retrograde cooling of the ureter and collecting system through infusion of ice-cold saline through a ureteral catheter during ablation. The authors found a lower risk of urinary leak in porcine kidneys.[53]

Although the techniques of percutaneous dissection and protective cooling have published success, cases are few in number. Risks of hydrodissection and CO_2 instillation include vascular injury, bowel laceration, and collecting system perforation, with unknown effects on the efficacy of RF treatment. In the authors' experience, we recommend that all tumors positioned within 1 cm of the bowel should be considered for a laparoscopic approach to provide definitive separation between the tumor and all vital structures.

MRI-guided technique

Lewin et al described the application of RFA using MRI guidance.[46] RF energy is delivered through custom-fabricated, MRI-compatible, 'cooled-tip' radiofrequency electrodes using a temperature-controlled system. Treatments are administered for 12 to 15 minutes at 90°C with real-time temperature monitoring of the RF lesion identified by changes in the MR enhancement patterns. If intraoperative imaging suggests incomplete treatment, the electrode is repositioned and additional RF cycles are performed. Follow-up is obtained through serial MRI scans to confirm the absence of persistent enhancement or radiographic recurrence. In the report two small, self-limited perinephric hematomas developed, but no other complications were identified. No tumor recurrences were detected at a mean follow-up of 25 months.

Laparoscopic-assisted technique

Lateral, medial, and anteriorly-oriented tumors inaccessible or perilous by radiologic percutaneous approaches are appropriate for laparoscopic mobilization of threatened structures, tumor identification, and percutaneous RFA treatment. Laparoscopy requires small port incisions, abdominal insufflation, and general anesthesia, but allows direct visualization of ablation needle placement.

The patient is placed in a modified-flank (45° tilt) position with the affected side elevated. The peritoneal cavity is accessed and the abdominal cavity is insufflated. Additional working ports are placed under direct vision. Typically only three ports are utilized: an umbilical 12 mm port for the placement of the laparoscopic ultrasound wand and two 5 mm ports for the operative laparoscope and dissecting instruments (Figure 7.13).

The line of Toldt is incised and the colon is reflected medially to expose the kidney. The tumor is localized under direct vision and laparoscopic ultrasound.

If peripheral temperature monitoring is performed, a minimum of three fiberoptic temperature sensors (Lumasense, Santa Clara, CA) are placed under ultrasound guidance at the peripheral (superior, inferior, lateral, medial) and deep margins of the tumor, 5 mm from the tumor–parenchymal interface (Figure 7.14). Using this method real-time temperature monitoring is available.

Tumor biopsies are obtained percutaneously prior to ablation. The RFA probe(s) is then positioned under direct visualization and ultrasound guidance, percutaneously between the previously placed temperature probes, directed toward the center of the tumor and advanced until the deep margin is reached with the probe tip. After the temperature sensors and ablation needle are properly positioned the RF cycle is initiated (Figure 7.15).

The ablation is complete after a specified time interval, temperature, or impedance goal is reached, or in the case of peripheral temperature monitoring when all thermistors reach the target temperature. Manipulation and alternate targeting of the RF probe and repeat application of RF energy may be necessary to achieve the target temperature at all monitored sites.

Basic science efficacy data

In the mid 1990s, RF energy was being used to ablate benign prostatic hypertrophy (TUNA).[54] In 1997, investigators began applying the technology to renal tissue.[38,55] During the initial experience with RFA

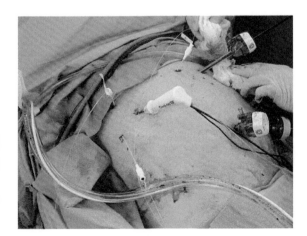

Figure 7.13 Laparoscopic-assisted RFA port and temperature fiber placement.

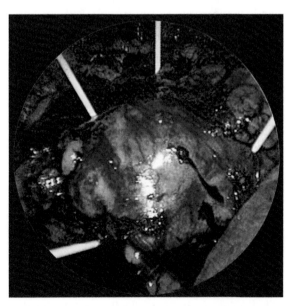

Figure 7.14 Laparoscopic-assisted RFA temperature fiber placement.

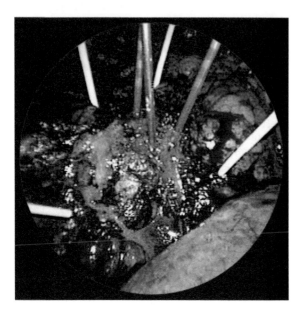

Figure 7.15 Laparoscopic-assisted RFA tumor surface.

several authors expressed concerns over the repeatability and reliability of ablation zones and demonstrating evidence of viable tumors cells with the ablated region.[56–58] Viable tissue examined by the authors may have actually represented tissue-processing effects from RFA damage (false-positives). Hsu et al were the first to describe the histologic appearance of RF lesions in a pig model. Percutaneous or laparoscopic RFA was performed on 11 pigs using a dry RFA electrode with 8–10 tines applied to normal renal parenchyma with an impedance-based system.[22] The changes seen on H&E staining included nuclear chromatin changes, loss of cell border integrity, and intracellular hemorrhage. Coagulation necrosis was demonstrated 3 days after treatment. Complete nuclear degeneration occurred by day 14 and all cellular architecture was lost by day 30. At 90 days inflammatory cells, hemorrhage, and necrotic tissue were all that remained.

If H&E histologic changes prove equivocal, NADH diaphorase staining is an alternative to determine cellular viability. NADH diaphorase reduces to NADH and a substrate and is present in all living cells. At death the NADH-reducing activity stops.[59] Follow-up studies to assess tissue viability with NADH-diaphorase staining supports complete tissue destruction following the RFA process.[60,61] Investigators have demonstrated stable H&E changes in the pig RFA model, contradicted with definitive evidence of cell kill on NADH-staining methods.[28,60,62] Marcovich et al also used NADH diaphorase staining after renal RFA in the pig model

and found that the central, definitively treated aspect of the tumors demonstrated no NADH activity, suggesting that NADH staining is a more accurate method to determine the viability of the tumors after RFA therapy.[60]

Histologic sections of RFA tumors also demonstrated thrombosed vessels.[28] Corwin et al investigated the effect of hilar clamping on lesion size and histology in a porcine model.[28] The renal hilum was clamped prior to RFA and then pigs were subsequently sacrificed immediately or up to 4 weeks later. H&E staining demonstrated preserved architecture immediately after ablation, but NADH diaphorase staining revealed total cellular death within the RFA lesion. The lesions in the clamped kidneys were larger than their unclamped counterparts, but adverse evidence of chronic pyelonephritis and one case of intraparenchymal hemorrhage were seen histologically in the clamped kidneys. Tan et al compared wet and dry RFA probes in a porcine model and looked at the specimens with H&E and NADH staining in the acute, subacute, and chronic settings. Post-RFA specimens removed immediately revealed preserved architecture, but absent NADH staining except in the glomeruli. Subacute and chronic specimens revealed necrosis and complete absence of NADH staining. Lesions were described as wedge-shaped consistent with vascular thrombosis.[62] Hilar clamping is not currently recommended in clinical practice for RFA treatment.

Polascik et al showed the renal medulla to be more sensitive to ablation than the renal cortex. Possible etiologies include a higher ion concentration in the medulla, resulting in a higher current and more intense heating.[55] Janzen et al determined that, although RFA does not spare the urothelium, there is solid evidence that RFA-treated urothelium regenerates over time.[63]

Comparisons of energy-delivery method and ablation probe configuration have been conducted through animal models.

Rehman et al[49] designed a study to compare 'wet' and 'dry' electrodes in a porcine model. Investigators examined 5 pigs treated with RF energy of 50 W at 500 kHz through single monopolar and bipolar electrode probes. Eighteen gauge needle electrodes with 2 cm of exposed tip were used for both circuit types. In the bipolar electrode the active and receiving portions were spaced 1 cm apart. Treatments were impedance regulated. RF energy was delivered for a 5-minute cycle and a total of 12 monopolar and 6 bipolar lesions were created. In 15 pigs a hollow 18 gauge needle with a 2 cm metal exposed tip was inserted into the renal parenchyma under ultrasound guidance for infusion of a gel substance. Infused liquids included hypertonic saline, ethanol, or acetic acid. RF energy was applied and the gel infusion continued at a rate of 2 ml/min. Both monopolar and bipolar energy were applied during the gel infusion. Three pigs were selected for heat-based RFA using a StarBurst XL (RITA Medical Systems, Mountain View, CA) multi-tined probe. The probe was placed under ultrasound guidance and deployed at 2.5 cm and 4.5 cm. Tissues were heated to >100°C for 10 minutes with real-time temperature management through thermocouples within the array. Six lesions were created. All kidneys were harvested at 1 week. Dry RF lesions displayed a loss of corticomedullary differentiation and lesions extending to but not violating the renal pelvis. A wedge-shaped area of coagulative necrosis was evident with a central zone of necrosis surrounded by a rim of inflammation. One monopolar and one bipolar lesion contained skip areas of viable tissue. Lesions obtained with simultaneous infusion of hypertonic saline were larger overall, with the monopolar lesions slightly larger than the bipolar lesions. Complete necrosis of the lesions with hypertonic saline and RF energy was appreciated microscopically. RF lesions obtained with both the ethanol infusion and acetic acid were similar and demonstrated complete necrosis. The acetic acid only group demonstrated complete necrosis without skip lesions. Lesions in the heat-based RF group demonstrated complete necrosis without skip lesions, and extension from the renal cortex into the renal pelvis.

Rehman et al also compared RFA lesions in pigs created with impedance- and temperatured-controlled systems with and without infusion of hypertonic saline. H&E staining showed viable cells after impedance-based RFA, but did not show viability after temperature-based or impedance-based RFA when using a 'wet' electrode. They concluded that dry impedance-based RFA may result in skip lesions.[49]

Gettman et al directly compared a temperature-controlled system with an impedance-based system in a pig model.[48] They concluded that both systems created uniform areas of ablation 2 cm in diameter, with cell death confirmed with NADH diaphorase staining.

Conclusions drawn from the animal studies state that cells may retain their normal architectural patterns for several weeks after ablation. Acute examined NADH staining can be positive in the glomeruli, but viability disappears subacutely. Wet RFA results in larger lesions than dry RFA.

Clinical efficacy data

Once efficacy and feasibility studies in animal models were complete, experience accumulated with RFA treatment in patients.

Zlotta et al performed the first RFA of a small renal tumor in 1997. The lesion was resected during a nephrectomy 1 week later. Investigators confirmed complete cellular necrosis with no evidence of viable tumor.[38] McGovern et al followed with a published case report of an 84-year-old male patient treated with percutaneous RFA for a suspicious 3.5 cm renal mass. Repeat imaging at 3 months revealed no enhancement of the lesion.[64]

The time-dependent histologic changes seen in animal models following RFA were also seen in a series of patients published by Walther et al.[65] The group performed RFA immediately before surgical excision in 4 patients with hereditary renal cell carcinoma. Pathologic evaluation reported loss of nuclear structure and non-visualization of the nucleoli in all tumors examined. Nuclear characteristics remained intact in the non-ablated group. Coagulative necrosis was not seen in the ablated specimens. Typically coagulative necrosis does not present until at least 48 hours following the ablation and becomes most pronounced at 7 days postoperatively.[66]

Marcovich et al treated tumors with RFA, immediately resected them, and then stained the tissue with both H&E and NADH diaphorase. The authors postulated that temperatures high enough to cause cellular death over time may not demonstrate acute changes in the cellular architecture. The group found that the histologic changes on H&E staining are not uniform and may be interspersed with areas of normal appearing renal tissue. NADH diaphorase is not included in these 'normal' appearing areas, supporting the idea that although they appear normal they are not viable.[60]

These studies illustrated the limitations to immediate pathologic evaluation after RFA and supported the idea that cellular damage continues to evolve after the lethal treatment is administered. Delayed pathologic examination is necessary to completely characterize the treated specimen.

This idea led Rendon et al to complete a study involving 4 patients treated with RFA then immediately resected by partial or radical nephrectomy. An additional 6 patients were treated with RFA and resected after a 7-day waiting period. Mean tumor size was 2.4 cm. An impedance-based system was used. Viable residual tumor volume was reported as 5–10% in 4 of 5 tumors in the RFA followed by immediate resection group. Between 5 and 10% viable residual tumor was also present in 3 of 6 patients in the delayed resection group.[57] This study raised questions about the accuracy of the probe targeting method (ultrasound) and the overall efficacy of the technique.

Michaels et al followed with a treatment of 20 tumors with RFA using a temperature-based electrode followed by partial nephrectomy. Each tumor was treated for 6 to 8 minutes, reaching a temperature of 90°C to 110°C. H&E staining revealed viable tumor cells in all specimens. Five specimens were stained for NADH activity, revealing a positive stain in 4 of 5 tumors indicating viable cells.[58]

Both studies question the completeness of RFA and its ability to destroy all targeted renal tumor. Failures in these studies may be attributable to flaws in the treatment technique. Impedance-based electrodes were not internally or externally cooled and may have prematurely developed carbonization at the electrode–tissue interface, resulting in limited energy delivery over shorter bursts. Size and geometry of the ablated lesion were not monitored during the procedure. Shorter ablation times with inadequate power were used in some cases.

Scientific evidence that externally and internally cooled RF probes allow more efficient, farther-reaching propagation of temperature led to investigations of new probe technologies in ablate and resect studies. Matlaga et al treated 10 patients with saline-cooled impedance-based RFA immediately prior to partial or radical nephrectomy; 200 W of power were used for a single 12-minute RFA cycle. Single probes were used for tumors <2 cm and cluster electrodes were used for tumors >2 cm. NADH diaphorase staining was performed; 8 of 10 tumors failed to reveal normal NADH diaphorase staining within the tumor. Of the two failures, one patient never achieved an adequate temperature for cellular kill (41°C) during the ablation, a result attributed to a heat-sink phenomenon. The other failure involved an 8 cm tumor which was felt to be too large to be treated effectively by RF. No complications related to treatment were noted.[56]

Success is defined in many series by radiographic follow-up imaging. Although animal studies suggest that a lack of enhancement on follow-up imaging suggests complete tumor destruction this idea has not been proven in humans.[57] Alternatives to demonstrate adequate tissue treatment include serial renal biopsy, but historically have a high rate of misinterpretation and sampling error. Follow-up data can also be obtained through serial contrasted CT scans. Lack of enhancement of tumor ablative success is defined by a rise in Hounsfield units of less than 10–20 HU (Figure 7.16).

Pavlovich et al[35] reported results of 24 tumors all <3 cm in 21 patients with either von Hippel–Lindau or hereditary papillary renal cancer. Treatments were performed percutaneously with a temperature-based 50 W generator. Two treatment cycles per tumor were completed with a target temperature of 70°C and times of 10–12 minutes each. A third cycle was performed if the tumor was larger than 3 cm or centrally located. Out of 24 tumors, 19 (79%) demonstrated no evidence of residual enhancement on CT scan 2 months later. Four of the 5 tumors with residual enhancement did not meet the target temperature during the treatment (>70°C). Four of the 5 failures were centrally-located tumors and

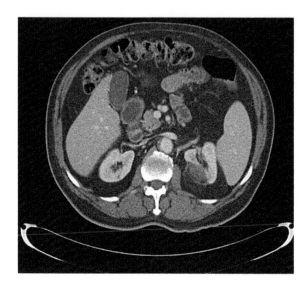

Figure 7.16 Postoperative CT scan following posterior RFA.

suspicious for a heat-sink phenomenon. These results show that radiographic results and clinical results are consistent; 40% of these lesions eventually developed residual enhancement at a follow-up of 24 months. All of these lesions were surgically removed and 9 of 10 of them had viable renal cell carcinoma.

Pavlovich et al performed a follow-up study using a 200 W cooled-tip RF electrode in 24 lesions <3 cm in size and found that only 1 lesion (4%) exhibited contrast enhancement at a follow-up of 1 year. The tumor was endophytic, centrally located, and difficult to access with the ablation probe.[35,67]

Mayo-Smith et al[68] used a combination of ultrasound and later CT-guided targeting of 38 lesions. Average renal mass size was 2.6 cm and success was defined as no enhancement on follow-up CT scans. A 200 W generator and cooled-tip electrode were used in single (12) and cluster (26) sessions. RFA treatment was successful in 31 of 32 (97%) after 1–2 ablation sessions. Some additional sessions were needed for larger masses and follow-up was an average of 9 months. Twenty-nine of 32 tumors were exophytic and none were centrally located.

RF treatment success may be influenced by tumor size and location, with endophytic or hilar lesions protected by the heat-sink effect of the renal vessels. Gervais et al reported 34 patients with 42 renal tumors treated with cooled-tip impedance-based systems. Single, cluster, and umbrella systems were all used. Follow-up was 13 months and success was documented in 100% of the exophytic tumors and parenchymal tumors. The success rate was reported as 86% for the 11 lesions with a component within close proximity to the renal sinus and thought to be a negative predictor of success. Only 5 of 11 tumors were successfully treated based on CT follow-up. These hilar tumors were hypothesized to be closer to the large vessels of the kidney and therefore thought to be associated with a heat sink that stole the heat away from the lesion. Smaller tumors (3 cm) faired better, with no failures in this group.[33] For the exophytic tumors, investigators found that 90% of tumors of 3 cm showed complete coagulation necrosis compared to 70% for tumors between 3.0 and 5.5 cm.[33]

Zagoria et al, in his series, found that success was extremely dependent on tumor size, but not on location, histology, or baseline renal insufficiency.[69] Authors found all tumors (11 of 11) <3 cm in their series to demonstrate a durable response to RF treatment.

Varkarakis et al reviewed their series of 56 renal lesions in 46 patients treated over a 4-year period.[70] RFA was performed under conscious sedation as an outpatient procedure, with both temperature and impedance control systems. Mean follow-up was 27 months. Imaging failures were seen in 6 tumors prior to 24 months (11%). Biopsy of the 6 lesions revealed 1 positive tumor. Failure to find viable tumor in the remaining 5 was postulated to result from a sampling error or false positive enhancement on CT imaging. Late failure (>24 months) was diagnosed in 3 tumors. All three lesions were endophytic and centrally located, possibly protected by a heat-sink phenomenon.

Su et al used percutaneous RFA to treat 35 tumors in 29 patients; 13 lesions had greater than 12 months of follow-up and 11 (85%) demonstrated no residual enhancement or growth. These authors suggested that ultrasound and CT may not be sufficient for real-time monitoring of the RFA lesions and cannot pinpoint the margin of the ablated tissue. They are advocates of real-time MRI for RFA targeting.[44]

Lewin et al[46] used MRI guidance to perform RFA in 10 renal lesions with an average follow-up of 25 months. Tumors preoperatively typically appeared as an area of high-signal intensity on T2-weighted images. Treatment was thought adequate when the T2-image changed to a low-signal intensity pattern. Post-treatment gadolinium-enhanced images were obtained to insure lack of contrast enhancement in those successfully treated lesions. Follow-up MRI scans have not revealed any residual enhancement or growth of the lesions.

Cadeddu et al[42,43] examined their experience with 109 renal lesions in 91 patients with almost all procedures performed under general anesthesia. A temperature control system was used and lesions were treated to 105°C (measured at the probe tip) for one or two cycles for 5–8 minutes. The treatment regimen was determined by the lesion size. Two patients (2%) demonstrated evidence of recurrence on 6-week follow-up CT scans and underwent repeat RFA treatment. One eventually developed a recurrence at 18 months postoperatively.

Mixed success in these studies emphasizes the need to perform RFA in a meticulous manner with excellent targeting and lesion monitoring. Full ablation should always be performed and multiple probes should be used when necessary to ablate completely beyond the interface between tumor and normal parenchyma in larger tumors. We advocate the use of peripheral temperature monitoring to ensure that lethal temperatures reach beyond the tumor margin.

ALTERNATIVE ABLATION TECHNIQUES

Cryoablation

Laparoscopic renal cryoablation has been performed since the mid-1990s with good intermediate results.[71,72] Cryoprobes are used to reach temperatures as low as −190°C through the Joule–Thompson effect of a compressed gas. In most systems, compressed argon is released and allowed to rapidly expand through a narrow diameter valve, causing temperatures in the adjacent tissue to fall well below experimental temperatures lethal to normal renal parenchyma as well as renal tumors. At temperatures below −19.4°C for normal renal parenchyma and −40°C for renal tumors cell death is achieved by a process of coagulative necrosis with subsequent fibrosis and scarring.[73] Renal cryoablation is applied through an open, laparoscopic, or percutaneous approach. The ice ball can be monitored with ultrasound, axial MRI, or CT.

Double freeze-thaw cycles are used to increase the size of the treatment lesion. Thawing can be passive or active, with helium gas used to expedite the process.

The edge of the ice ball typically reaches a temperature of 0°C. At this temperature both normal renal parenchyma and cancer tissue will survive, therefore it is necessary to extend the treatment margin to approximately 1 cm beyond the tumor edge. This 1 cm treatment margin creates an 'indeterminant' zone where the outer few millimeters of the ice ball are non-ablative and overlap with normal renal parenchyma.[74] Although most of the ice ball growth occurs in the first 5 minutes, studies have shown that it takes approximately 20 minutes to reach a steady state.[75] Therefore, sustained freeze cycles greater than 20 minutes are recommended.

When cryoablation probes are removed at the conclusion of the case, hemostatic agents are usually necessary. Thrombin-derived and other matrix scaffold materials are applied directly to the ablation tract.

Reported cryoablation series demonstrate an overall persistence or recurrence rate of 4.6% and a complication rate of 10.6%.[71]

High-intensity focused ultrasound

High-intensity focused ultrasound (HIFU) energy is created from piezoelectric elements that are focused with an acoustic lens or parabolic reflector.[76] The HIFU energy is absorbed by the tissue and results in a focal heat production that is sufficient to denature intracellular proteins and cause coagulative necrosis. Tissue cavitation and vibration occur at 5000–20 000 W/cm^2 and can be visualized in real time with ultrasound. When attempting to apply ultrasound energy from outside the body, limitations in targeting occur due to lesion movement with respiration, interposed organs or overlying ribs, and poor visualization of the tumor. Laparoscopic probes capable of delivering HIFU energy have been developed, but remove the true advantage of this therapy, approaching the lesion transcutaneously without the need for incisions in a truly minimally invasive method.

Data supporting the efficacy of HIFU in the treatment of renal tumors are limited. Kohrmann et al[76] reported the treatment of 3 renal tumors with HIFU. The 2 lower pole tumors in the series were smaller on repeat imaging, but the upper pole tumor remained the same size. The ultrasound energy was thought to be absorbed by the overlying ribs. Marberger et al[77] treated 16 patients. Immediate surgical excision was performed in 14 patients; tumor necrosis secondary to HIFU-applied energy was identified in 15–35% of the targeted area in 9 patients; 5 patients demonstrated skin erythema.

A phase II clinical trial at Churchill Hospital, Oxford, UK involved 4 patients with renal tumors treated with HIFU. Surgical excision was performed 6 weeks after HIFU therapy in 3 of 4 patients, with no conclusive evidence of ablation in these 3 patients.

Wu et al[78] treated 13 patients with renal tumors; 10 patients were treated palliatively for advanced or metastatic disease and 3 were treated with curative intent for local disease. Palliation results were reported only with tumor volume decreasing by 58% and one lesion disappearing completely radiographically.

Results appear mixed at this time, but HIFU technology and techniques continue to progress and may prove more efficacious in the future.

COMPLICATIONS

Laparoscopic and radiographically-guided percutaneous RFA is offered to patients seeking a minimally invasive approach to therapy of their renal lesions. Although patients and clinicians expect minimal morbidity, complications are still possible.

Uzzo and Novick[79] reviewed the literature from 1980 to 2000 and found a complication rate for nephron-sparing procedures (the majority were parital nephrectomies) ranging from 4 to 30%, with an average of 13.7%. To become an accepted form of nephron-sparing therapy, RFA must demonstrate equivalent oncologic efficacy with lower complication rates.

The majority of complications reported in the literature are minor and include subcapsular or perinephric hematomas that do not require treatment. Few others require definitive therapy. Biliary fistula has been reported in a porcine model.[49] Uretero-pelvic junction (UPJ) obstructions have been described requiring pyeloplasty in one and nephrectomy secondary to pain and loss of renal function in the other.[58,80] A case of skin metastasis to an electrode site has occurred.[68]

Transient acute oliguric renal failure in a patient with a solitary kidney has been reported. The patient had 7 renal lesions in the solitary kidney, 6 were treated with RF and 1 with a partial nephrectomy.[81]

A multi-institutional review of complications of cryoablation and RFA was performed.[82] Eleven complications were seen in 133 cases (8.3%) of RFA; 8 complications were listed as minor, requiring no intervention, and 3 were considered major. Minor complications were described as pain and paresthesias at the probe puncture site, and transiently increased serum creatinine. Major complications included an ileus, a UPJ obstruction that ultimately led to renal loss and nephrectomy, and a urinary leak.

The 8.3% complication rate is certainly comparable to the 13.7% overall experience with partial nephrectomy, and is more impressive considering that many RFA patients were deemed inappropriate for more invasive surgical therapies.

POSTABLATION MONITORING AND IMAGING

After RFA treatment, tumors are monitored by contrasted CT or MRI with no lesion enhancement and no evidence of growth indicative of a treatment success. Viable tumor should display persistent or recurrent enhancement, with cutoff values ranging from 5 to 20 HU units of change pre- to postcontrast, based on author preference. Long-term experience with following ablated tumors radiographically is lacking and optimal surveillance intervals are yet to be determined. Unlike cryoablated lesions, RFA lesions tend not to shrink in size. Matsumoto et al described the typical characteristics of the radiofrequency ablated mass. These characteristics include a non-enhancing wedge-shaped lesion with frequently a thin rim of fat between the lesion and the normal parenchyma. Exophytic tumors tend to retain their pre-ablation shape and size.[83]

Imaging characteristics can change at any time and a regimented follow-up protocol is encouraged in all patients. Recurrences have been documented as late as 31 months.

SUMMARY AND CONCLUSION

Precise targeting of ablative energy and an assurance that adequate lesion treatment has occurred are critical challenges facing minimally invasive therapy for renal cell carcinoma. Energy targeting is greatly enhanced through imaging modalities such as ultrasound, MRI, and CT scanning to assist needle placement or energy delivery to the optimal location for maximal effectiveness. When vital structures obscure access to the renal lesion, laparoscopic mobilization of these structures with direct visualization of the tumor can increase the likelihood of ablation success and minimize complication risk. Monitoring the size and geometry of the ablation lesion ensures that the outermost reaches of the renal tumor have been completely treated. Authors have described contrasted ultrasound and MRI for real-time imaging of the ablative lesion. We advocate the use of real-time temperature measurement with fiber-optic sensors placed at the tumor periphery. Independent of the ablation type or control method, when sustained lethal temperatures are recorded at the tumor margins the clinician can be confident that the treatment is complete.

Ablative therapies are attractive due to their minimal impact on patient quality of life. Patients spend less time in hospital, require less pain medication, and resume their normal activity level sooner than traditional surgical approaches to renal cell carcinoma. Although ablative therapies show promise of efficacy, they must be evaluated with long-term follow-up before they are considered the standard of oncologic care. Safety profiles thus far are excellent and, as technology and techniques advance, ablative therapies gain more widespread use and acceptance.

REFERENCES

1. Jemal A, Siegel R, Ward E et al. Cancer statistics, 2006. CA Cancer J Clin 2006; 56: 106.
2. Luciani LG, Cestari R, Tallarigo C. Incidental renal cell carcinoma – age and stage characterization and clinical implications: study of 1092 patients (1982–1997). Urology 2000; 56: 58.
3. Hafez KS, Fergany AF, Novick AC. Nephron sparing surgery for localized renal cell carcinoma: impact of tumor size on patient survival, tumor recurrence and TNM staging. J Urol 1999; 162: 1930.
4. Pantuck AJ, Zisman A, Rauch MK et al. Incidental renal tumors. Urology 2000; 56: 190.
5. Dechet CB, Sebo T, Farrow G et al. Prospective analysis of intraoperative frozen needle biopsy of solid renal masses in adults. J Urol 1999; 162: 1282.
6. Novick AC. Laparoscopic and partial nephrectomy. Clin Cancer Res 2004; 10: 6322S.
7. Fergany AF, Hafez KS, Novick AC. Long-term results of nephron sparing surgery for localized renal cell carcinoma: 10-year followup. J Urol 2000; 163: 442.
8. Lee CT, Katz J, Shi W et al. Surgical management of renal tumors 4 cm or less in a contemporary cohort. J Urol 2000; 163: 730.
9. Finelli A, Gill IS. Laparoscopic partial nephrectomy: contemporary technique and results. Urol Oncol 2004; 22: 139.
10. Lau WY, Leung TW, Yu SC et al. Percutaneous local ablative therapy for hepatocellular carcinoma: a review and look into the future. Ann Surg 2003; 237: 171.
11. Lencioni R, Crocetti L, Cioni D et al. Percutaneous radiofrequency ablation of hepatic colorectal metastases: technique, indications, results, and new promises. Invest Radiol 2004; 39: 689.
12. Mirza A, Fornage B. Radiofrequency ablation of solid tumors. Cancer J 2001; 7.
13. Zagoria RJ, Chen MY, Kavanagh PV et al. Radio frequency ablation of lung metastases from renal cell carcinoma. J Urol 2001; 166: 1827.
14. Gervais DA, Arellano RS, Mueller PR. Percutaneous radiofrequency ablation of nodal metastases. Cardiovasc Intervent Radiol 2002; 25: 547.
15. McAchran SE, Lesani OA, Resnick MI. Radiofrequency ablation of renal tumors: past, present, and future. Urology 2005; 66: 15.
16. Leveillee RJ, Hoey MF. Radiofrequency interstitial tissue ablation: wet electrode. J Endourol 2003; 17: 563.
17. Beer E. Removal of neoplasms of the urinary bladder: a new method, employing high frequency (Oudin) currents. JAMA 1910.
18. McCarthy J. A new type of observation and operating cysto-urethroscope. J Urol 1923; 10: 519.
19. Pennes H. Analysis of tissue and arterial blood temperatures in the resting forearm. J Appl Physiol 1948; 1: 93.
20. Organ LW. Electrophysiologic principles of radiofrequency lesion making. Appl Neurophysiol 1976; 39: 69.
21. Mulier S, Miao Y, Mulier P et al. Electrodes and multiple electrode systems for radiofrequency ablation: a proposal for updated terminology. Eur Radiol 2005; 15: 798.
22. Hsu TH, Fidler ME, Gill IS. Radiofrequency ablation of the kidney: acute and chronic histology in porcine model. Urology 2000; 56: 872.
23. Crowley JD, Shelton J, Iverson AJ et al. Laparoscopic and computed tomography-guided percutaneous radiofrequency ablation of renal tissue: acute and chronic effects in an animal model. Urology 2001; 57: 976.
24. Lele P. Thresholds and mechanisms of ultrasonic damage to organized animal tissues. Presented at the Symposium on Biological Effects and Characterizations of Ultrasound Sources, Rockville, MD, 1977.
25. Djavan B, Zlotta AR, Susani M et al. Transperineal radiofrequency interstitial tumor ablation of the prostate: correlation of magnetic resonance imaging with histopathologic examination. Urology 1997; 50: 986.
26. Bhowmick S, Swanlund DJ, Coad JE et al. Evaluation of thermal therapy in a prostate cancer model using a wet electrode radiofrequency probe. J Endourol 2001; 15: 629.
27. McGahan JP, Brock JM, Tesluk H et al. Hepatic ablation with use of radio-frequency electrocautery in the animal model. J Vasc Intervent Radiol 1992; 3: 291.

28. Corwin TS, Lindberg G, Traxer O et al. Laparoscopic radiofrequency thermal ablation of renal tissue with and without hilar occlusion. J Urol 2001; 166: 281.

29. Chang I, Mikityansky I, Wray-Cahen D et al. Effects of perfusion on radiofrequency ablation in swine kidneys. Radiology 2004; 231: 500.

30. Haines DE, Watson DD. Tissue heating during radiofrequency catheter ablation: a thermodynamic model and observations in isolated perfused and superfused canine right ventricular free wall. Pacing Clin Electrophysiol 1989; 12: 962.

31. Hoey MF, Mulier PM, Leveillee RJ et al. Transurethral prostate ablation with saline electrode allows controlled production of larger lesions than conventional methods. J Endourol 1997; 11: 279.

32. Goldberg SN, Gazelle GS, Solbiati L et al. Radiofrequency tissue ablation: increased lesion diameter with a perfusion electrode. Acad Radiol 1996; 3: 636.

33. Gervais DA, McGovern FJ, Arellano RS et al. Renal cell carcinoma: clinical experience and technical success with radiofrequency ablation of 42 tumors. Radiology 2003; 226: 417.

34. Pereira PL, Trubenbach J, Schenk M et al. Radiofrequency ablation: in vivo comparison of four commercially available devices in pig livers. Radiology 2004; 232: 482.

35. Pavlovich CP, Walther MM, Choyke PL et al. Percutaneous radio frequency ablation of small renal tumors: initial results. J Urol 2002; 167: 10.

36. Poon RT, Fan ST, Tsang FH et al. Locoregional therapies for hepatocellular carcinoma: a critical review from the surgeon's perspective. Ann Surg 2002; 235: 466.

37. Goldberg SN, Gazelle GS. Radiofrequency tissue ablation: physical principles and techniques for increasing coagulation necrosis. Hepatogastroenterology 2001; 48: 359.

38. Zlotta AR, Wildschutz T, Raviv G et al. Radiofrequency interstitial tumor ablation (RITA) is a possible new modality for treatment of renal cancer: ex vivo and in vivo experience. J Endourol 1997; 11: 251.

39. Nakada SY, Jerde TJ, Warner TF et al. Bipolar radiofrequency ablation of the kidney: comparison with monopolar radiofrequency ablation. J Endourol 2003; 17: 927.

40. Lee FT Jr, Haemmerich D, Wright AS et al. Multiple probe radiofrequency ablation: pilot study in an animal model. J Vasc Intervent Radiol 2003; 14: 1437.

41. Johnson DB, Duchene DA, Taylor GD et al. Contrast-enhanced ultrasound evaluation of radiofrequency ablation of the kidney: reliable imaging of the thermolesion. J Endourol 2005; 19: 248.

42. Johnson DB, Duchene DA, Taylor GD, Pearle MS, Cadeddu JU. Contrast-enhanced ultrasound evaluation of radiofrequency ablation of the kidney: reliable imaging of the thermolesion. J Endourol 2005; 19(2): 248–52.

43. Matsumoto ED, Johnson DB, Ogan K et al. Shor-term efficacy of temperature-based radiofrequency ablation of small renal tumors. Urology 2005; 65(5): 877–81.

44. Su LM, Jarrett TW, Chan DY et al. Percutaneous computed tomography-guided radiofrequency ablation of renal masses in high surgical risk patients: preliminary results. Urology 2003; 61: 26.

45. Merkle EM, Shonk JR, Duerk JL et al. MR-guided RF thermal ablation of the kidney in a porcine model. AJR Am J Roentgenol 1999; 173: 645.

46. Lewin JS, Nour SG, Connell CF et al. Phase II clinical trial of interactive MR imaging-guided interstitial radiofrequency thermal ablation of primary kidney tumors: initial experience. Radiology 2004; 232: 835.

47. Carey R. Radiofrequency ablation of renal tumors between 3 and 5 centimeters using direct, real time temperature monitoring. J Endourol 2007.

48. Gettman MT, Lotan Y, Corwin TS et al. Radiofrequency coagulation of renal parenchyma: comparison of effects of energy generators on treatment efficacy. J Endourol 2002; 16: 83.

49. Rehman J, Landman J, Lee D et al. Needle-based ablation of renal parenchyma using microwave, cryoablation, impedance- and temperature-based monopolar and bipolar radiofrequency, and liquid and gel chemoablation: laboratory studies and review of the literature. J Endourol 2004; 18: 83.

50. Rendon RA, Gertner MR, Sherar MD et al. Development of a radiofrequency based thermal therapy technique in an in vivo porcine model for the treatment of small renal masses. J Urol 2001; 166: 292.

51. Farrell MA, Charboneau JW, Callstrom MR et al. Paranephric water instillation: a technique to prevent bowel injury during percutaneous renal radiofrequency ablation. Am J Roentgenol 2003; 181: 1315.

52. Yamakado K, Nakatsuka A, Akeboshi M et al. Percutaneous radiofrequency ablation of liver neoplasms adjacent to the gastrointestinal tract after balloon catheter interposition. J Vasc Intervent Radiol 2003; 14: 1183.

53. Margulis V, Matsumoto ED, Taylor G et al. Retrograde renal cooling during radio frequency ablation to protect from renal collecting system injury. J Urol 2005; 174: 350.

54. Ramon J, Lynch TH, Eardley I et al. Transurethral needle ablation of the prostate for the treatment of benign prostatic hyperplasia: a collaborative multicentre study. Br J Urol 1997; 80: 128.

55. Polascik TJ, Hamper U, Lee BR et al. Ablation of renal tumors in a rabbit model with interstitial saline-augmented radiofrequency energy: preliminary report of a new technology. Urology 1999; 53: 465.

56. Matlaga BR, Zagoria RJ, Woodruff RD et al. Phase II trial of radio frequency ablation of renal cancer: evaluation of the kill zone. J Urol 2002; 168: 2401.

57. Rendon RA, Kachura JR, Sweet JM et al. The uncertainty of radio frequency treatment of renal cell carcinoma: findings at immediate and delayed nephrectomy. J Urol 2002; 167: 1587.

58. Michaels MJ, Rhee HK, Mourtzinos AP et al. Incomplete renal tumor destruction using radio frequency interstitial ablation. J Urol 2002; 168: 2406.

59. Neumann RA, Knobler RM, Pieczkowski F et al. Enzyme histochemical analysis of cell viability after argon laser-induced coagulation necrosis of the skin. J Am Acad Dermatol 1991; 25: 991.

60. Marcovich R, Aldana JP, Morgenstern N et al. Optimal lesion assessment following acute radio frequency ablation of porcine kidney: cellular viability or histopathology? J Urol 2003; 170: 1370.

61. Johnson DB, Cadeddu JA. Radiofrequency interstitial tumor ablation: dry electrode. J Endourol 2003; 17: 557.

62. Tan BJ, El-Hakim A, Morgenstern N et al. Comparison of laparoscopic saline infused to dry radio frequency ablation of renal tissue: evolution of histological infarct in the porcine model. J Urol 2004; 172: 2007.

63. Janzen NK, Perry KT, Han KR et al. The effects of intentional cryoablation and radio frequency ablation of renal tissue involving the collecting system in a porcine model. J Urol 2005; 173: 1368.

64. McGovern FJ, Wood BJ, Goldberg SN et al. Radio frequency ablation of renal cell carcinoma via image guided needle electrodes. J Urol 1999; 161: 599.

65. Walther MC, Shawker TH, Libutti SK et al. A phase 2 study of radio frequency interstitial tissue ablation of localized renal tumors. J Urol 2000; 163: 1424.

66. Schulman CC, Zlotta AR. Transurethral needle ablation of the prostate (TUNA). A new treatment of benign prostatic hyperplasia using interstitial radiofrequency energy. J Urol (Paris) 1995; 101: 33.

67. Hwang JJ, Walther MM, Pautler SE et al. Radio frequency ablation of small renal tumors: intermediate results. J Urol 2004; 171: 1814.

68. Mayo-Smith WW, Dupuy DE, Parikh PM et al. Imaging-guided percutaneous radiofrequency ablation of solid renal masses: techniques and outcomes of 38 treatment sessions in 32 consecutive patients. AJR Am J Roentgenol 2003; 180: 1503.

69. Zagoria RJ, Hawkins AD, Clark PE et al. Percutaneous CT-guided radiofrequency ablation of renal neoplasms: factors influencing success. AJR Am J Roentgenol 2004; 183: 201.

70. Varkarakis IM, Allaf ME, Inagaki T et al. Percutaneous radio frequency ablation of renal masses: results at a 2-year mean followup. J Urol 2005; 174: 456.

71. Lee DI, McGinnis DE, Feld R et al. Retroperitoneal laparoscopic cryoablation of small renal tumors: intermediate results. Urology 2003; 61: 83.

72. Gill IS, Novick AC, Meraney AM et al. Laparoscopic renal cryoablation in 32 patients. Urology 2000; 56: 748.

73. Chosy SG, Nakada SY, Lee FT Jr et al. Monitoring renal cryosurgery: predictors of tissue necrosis in swine. J Urol 1998; 159: 1370.

74. Weld KJ, Landman J. Comparison of cryoablation, radiofrequency ablation and high-intensity focused ultrasound for treating small renal tumours. BJU Int 2005; 96: 1224.

75. Gage AA. Cryosurgery in the treatment of cancer. Surg Gynecol Obstet 1992; 174: 73.

76. Kohrmann KU, Michel MS, Gaa J et al. High intensity focused ultrasound as noninvasive therapy for multilocal renal cell carcinoma: case study and review of the literature. J Urol 2002; 167: 2397.

77. Marberger M, Schatzl G, Cranston D et al. Extracorporeal ablation of renal tumours with high-intensity focused ultrasound. BJU Int 2005; 95(Suppl 2): 52.

78. Wu F, Wang ZB, Chen WZ et al. Preliminary experience using high intensity focused ultrasound for the treatment of patients with advanced stage renal malignancy. J Urol 2003; 170: 2237–40.

79. Uzzo RG, Novick AC. Nephron sparing surgery for renal tumors: indications, techniques and outcomes. J Urol 2001; 166: 6.

80. Johnson DB, Saboorian MH, Duchene DA et al. Nephrectomy after radiofrequency ablation-induced ureteropelvic junction obstruction: potential complication and long-term assessment of ablation adequacy. Urology 2003; 62: 351.

81. Ogan K, Cadeddu JA, Sagalowsky AI. Radio frequency ablation induced acute renal failure. J Urol 2002; 168: 186.

82. Johnson DB, Solomon SB, Su LM et al. Defining the complications of cryoablation and radio frequency ablation of small renal tumors: a multi-institutional review. J Urol 2004; 172: 874.

83. Matsumoto ED, Watumull L, Johnson DB et al. The radiographic evolution of radio frequency ablated renal tumors. J Urol 2004; 172: 45.

8

Laparoscopic partial nephrectomy

Saleh Binsaleh and Anil Kapoor

INTRODUCTION

In 1991 Clayman et al described the first successful laparoscopic nephrectomy.[1] Since that time, laparoscopic radical nephrectomy for renal tumors has been routinely performed in select patients worldwide. During this period, 'elective' open partial nephrectomy has established itself as an efficacious therapeutic approach in the treatment of small renal masses[2] similar to that of radical nephrectomy in select patients with a small renal tumor. At the same time the widespread use of contemporary imaging techniques has resulted in an increased detection of small incidental renal tumors, in which the management, during the past decade, has been trended away from radical nephrectomy toward nephron-conserving surgery. In 1993 successful laparoscopic partial nephrectomy (LPN) was first reported in a porcine model,[3] while Winfield et al reported the first human LPN in 1993.[4] From that time, several centers in the world have developed laparoscopic techniques for partial nephrectomy through retroperitoneal or transperitoneal approaches. In the beginning, only small, peripheral, exophytic tumors were wedge excised, but with experience, larger, infiltrating tumors have been managed similarly.[5]

LPN combines the advances and benefits of nephron-sparing surgery and laparoscopy to offer a decreased morbidity inherent to laparoscopy while preserving the renal function offered by partial nephrectomy.

Technical difficulty in LPN is encountered when securing renal hypothermia, renal parenchymal hemostasis, pelvicalyceal reconstruction, and parenchymal renorrhaphy by pure laparoscopic techniques. Nevertheless, ongoing advances in laparoscopic techniques and operator skills have allowed the development of a reliable technique of laparoscopic partial nephrectomy, duplicating the established principles and technical steps underpinning open partial nephrectomy.

In this chapter we evaluate the role of LPN in the nephron-sparing armamentarium.

INDICATIONS AND CONTRAINDICATIONS

Partial nephrectomy is frequently done for benign and malignant renal conditions. In the setting of malignant renal diseases, this is indicated in situations where radical nephrectomy would leave the patient anephric due to bilateral renal tumors or unilateral tumor and compromised or at risk the other side. Some investigators also defined the role of elective PN in patients with unilateral renal tumors and normal contralateral kidneys.[6]

Due to its technical limitations, LPN was initially reserved for select patients with a small, peripheral, superficial, exophytic tumor, but as laparoscopic experience increased, the indications were carefully expanded to select patients with more complex tumors, such as tumor invading deeply into the parenchyma up to the collecting system or renal sinus, completely intrarenal tumor, tumor abutting the renal hilum, tumor in a solitary kidney, or tumor substantial enough to require heminephrectomy. It is important to stress the fact that LPN for these complex tumors is performed in the setting of a compromised or threatened total renal function wherein nephron preservation is an important goal.

General contraindications to abdominal laparoscopic surgery are applied to LPN. Specific absolute contraindications to LPN include bleeding diathesis (such as renal failure induced platelet dysfunction and blood thinners), renal vein thrombus, multiple renal tumors, and aggressive locally advanced disease. Morbid obesity and a history of prior renal surgery may prohibitively increase the technical complexity of the procedure and should be considered a relative contraindication for LPN.

Overall, the ultimate decision to proceed with LPN should be based on the tumor characteristics and the surgeon's skill and experience with such an approach.

PREOPERATIVE PREPARATION

Preoperative evaluation includes a complete blood count, renal function test, chest X-ray, and computed tomography angiogram of the abdomen to clearly assess the vascular anatomy. Renal scintigraphy is obtained if there is a question about the global renal function. Clearance for fitness for major abdominal surgery is obtained whenever indicated.

We routinely cross-match 4 units of packed red blood cells on demand. Mechanical bowel preparation of one bottle of magnesium citrate is given the evening before the surgery, and intravenous prophylactic antibiotics are given upon calling the patient to the operating room.

OPERATIVE TECHNIQUE

A substantive LPN entails renal hilar control, transection of major intrarenal vessels, controlled entry into and repair of the collecting system, control of parenchymal blood vessels, and renal parenchymal reconstruction, all usually under the 'gun of warm ischemia.' As such, significant experience in the minimally invasive environment, including expertise with time-sensitive intracorporeal suturing, is essential.

LPN can be approached either transperitoneally (our preferred approach) or retroperitoneally based on the surgeon's experience and the tumor location. The transperitoneal approach is usually chosen for anterior, anterolateral, lateral, and upper-pole apical tumors. Retroperitoneal laparoscopy is reserved for posterior or posterolaterally located tumors.

After induction of general anesthesia, a Foley catheter and nasogastric tube are placed prior to patient positioning. Cystoscopy and ureteral catheter placement are performed if preoperative imaging indicates a risk of collecting system violation during resection of the lesion (a requirement for intraparenchymal resection greater than 1.5 cm or tumor abutting the collecting system). Although many laparoscopists prefer to place their patients at a 45 to 60° angle in the flank position, we prefer to place our patients undergoing renal surgery in the lateral flank position at 90°. This provides excellent access to the hilum and allows the bowel and spleen (on the left side) to fall off the renal hilum during procedures complicated by bowel distention.

Laparoscopic surgery is performed using a transperitoneal approach with a Veress needle, or directly using the Optiview trocar system to attain pneumoperitoneum. Three to four ports (including two 10–12 mm ports) are routinely placed in our technique. Exposure of the kidney and the hilar dissection are performed using a J-hook electrocautery suction probe or by using the ultrasound energy-based harmonic shears (Ethicon Endo-surgery). This is done by reflecting the mesocolon along the line of Toldt, leaving Gerota's fascia intact. Mobilizing the kidney within this fascia, the ureter is retracted laterally, and cephalad dissection is carried out along the psoas muscle leading to the renal hilum. Once the tumor is localized, we dissect the Gerota's fascia and defat the kidney, leaving only the perinephric fat overlying the tumor (Figure 8.1). Intraoperative ultrasonography with a Philips Entos LAP 9–5 linear array transducer (Philips) can be used to aid in tumor localization if it is not exophytic or if the tumor is deep into the renal parenchyma. A laparoscopic vascular clamp (Karl Storz) is placed around both the renal artery and the renal vein (without separation of the vessels) for hilar control in cases associated with central masses and heminephrectomy procedures, as described by Gill et al[7] (Figures 8.2–8.4). Conversely, during a retroperitoneoscopic partial nephrectomy, the renal artery and vein are dissected separately to prepare for placement of bulldog clamps on the renal artery and vein individually. Mannitol may be used (0.5 g/kg intravenously) prior to hilar clamping or renal hypothermia. Resection of renal parenchyma is performed with cold scissor (Figures 8.5–8.10), and the specimen is retrieved using a 10-cm laparoscopic EndoCatch bag (US Surgical Corporation, Norwalk, Connecticut) and sent for frozen section analysis (sometimes with an excisional biopsy from the base) to determine the resection margin status (Figures 8.11 and 8.12).

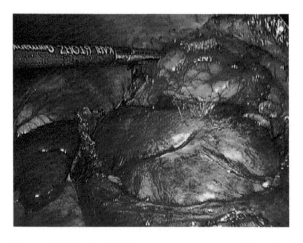

Figure 8.1 Defatted kidney, except area overlying the tumor.

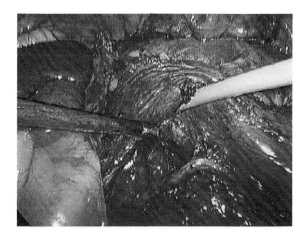

Figure 8.2 Exposed renal hilum.

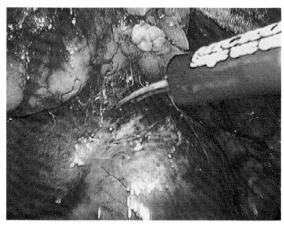

Figure 8.5 Tumor resection using the cold scissor.

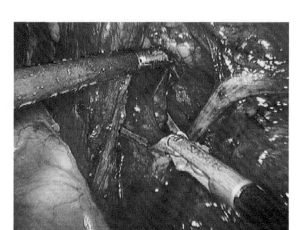

Figure 8.3 Exposed hilum ready for clamping.

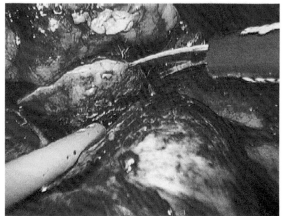

Figure 8.6 Continued tumor resection with surrounding normal parenchyma.

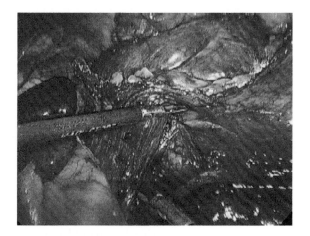

Figure 8.4 Clamped renal hilum.

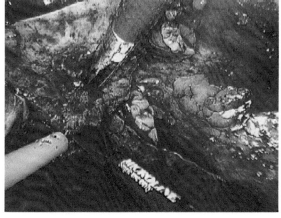

Figure 8.7 Continued tumor resection.

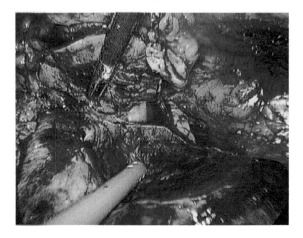

Figure 8.8 Completely detached tumor.

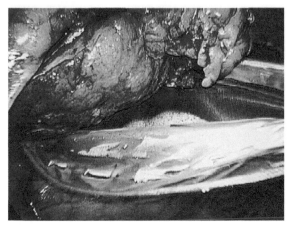

Figure 8.11 Tumor entrapment in an Endocatch bag.

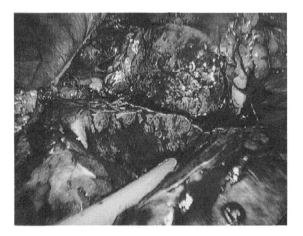

Figure 8.9 Completely detached tumor with good surrounding parenchyma.

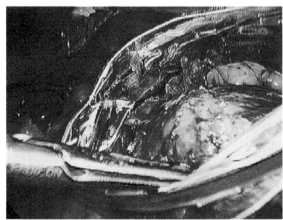

Figure 8.12 Tumor completely entrapped.

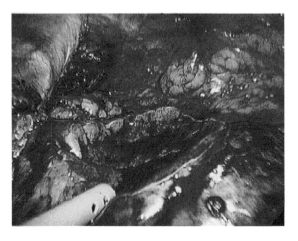

Figure 8.10 Tumor bed.

Hemostasis is accomplished using intracorporeal suturing, argon beam coagulator, and fibrin sealant (Tisseel®, Baxter, Vienna, Austria) application in a manner previously described by others[8–11] (Figures 8.13–8.20). Intravenous injection of indigo carmine dye is used to delineate any collecting system violation, or retrograde injection of this dye via a ureteric catheter if it was inserted perioperatively. Any identifiable leak in the collecting system is oversewn with 40 absorbable sutures using the freehand intracorporeal laparoscopic technique. If the collecting system is entered, ureteral stenting additional to a Jackson–Pratt percutanous drain placement is routinely performed (Figure 8.21). Specific figure-of-eight sutures are placed at the site of visible individual transected intrarenal vessels using a CT-1 needle and 20 Vicryl suture. Parenchymal closure is achieved by placing prefashioned rolled tubes or packets of oxidized cellulose

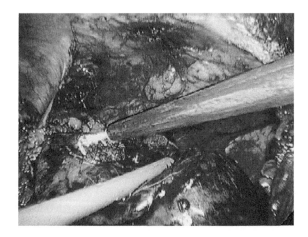

Figure 8.13 Argon beam coagulator for bed hemostasis.

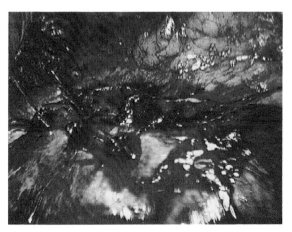

Figure 8.16 Completed sutures with Lapra-TY on both ends.

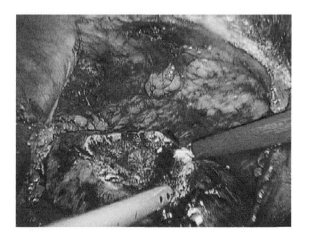

Figure 8.14 Argon beam coagulator for bed hemostasis.

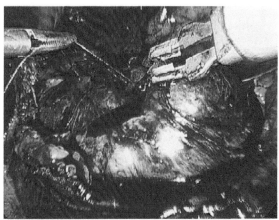

Figure 8.17 Parenchymal suturing with Lapra-TY.

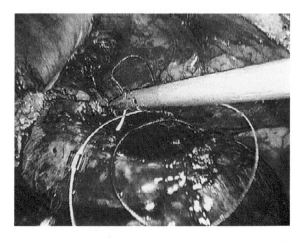

Figure 8.15 Parenchymal intracorporeal suturing with Lapra-TY at one end.

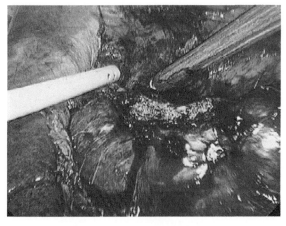

Figure 8.18 Hemostasis with argon beam coagulator after hilar unclamping.

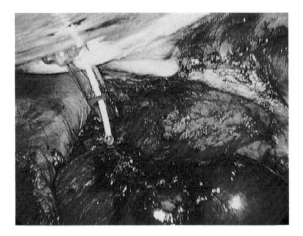

Figure 8.19 Fibrin sealant (Tisseel) applied over the sutured bed.

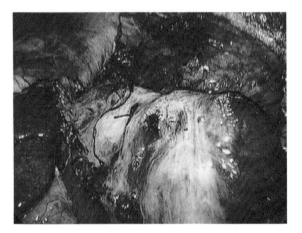

Figure 8.20 Completed Tisseel.

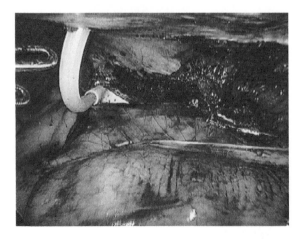

Figure 8.21 Percutanous drain around the operated site.

sheets (Surgicel®, Ethicon) into the parenchymal defect. Braided 20 absorbable sutures are used to bolster the sheets into position, and fibrin glue is applied over the operative site using a laparoscopic applicator.

Recently we modified our parenchymal repair into using multiple interrupted 20 absorbable sutures and securing them in position using absorbable polydioxanone polymer suture clips (Lapra-TY®, Ethicon, Endosurgery). Placing one Lapra-TY clip to the end of the suture then another one to the opposite side after compressing the kidney achieves this (Figures 8.15–8.17). This modification has resulted in a significant reduction of our warm ischemia time that was consumed primarily by intracorporeal suturing. Once renorrhaphy is completed, the vascular clamp is released, and the complete hemostasis and renal revascularization is confirmed. Whenever possible, the perinephric fat and Gerota's fascia is re-approximated. We extract the resected tumor along with its containing bag through a small extension of the lowermost abdominal port site incision. Laparoscopic exit under direct vision is performed once the 10–12 mm ports are closed.

ISSUES IN LAPAROSCOPIC PARTIAL NEPHRECTOMY

Warm ischemia and renal hypothermia

The highly differentiated cellular architecture of the kidney is dependent on the primarily aerobic renal metabolism. As such, the kidney is acutely vulnerable to the anaerobic insult conferred by warm ischemia. The severity of renal injury and its reversibility are directly proportional to the period of warm ischemia time (WIT) imposed on the unprotected kidney. Previous studies have demonstrated that recovery of renal function is complete within minutes after 10 minutes of warm ischemia, within hours after 20 minutes, within 3 to 9 days after 30 minutes, usually within weeks after 60 minutes, and incomplete or absent after 120 minutes of warm ischemia.[12–14] For this reason it is widely accepted to limit the warm renal ischemia time during partial nephrectomy to periods of 30 minutes or less. If the warm ischemia is anticipated to last greater than 30 minutes, renal hypothermia is advisable before proceeding with partial nephrectomy. However, this guideline was based on studies that were either not designed to address the limits of WIT specifically or did not assess the long-term recovery of renal function. In addition, many used crude methods of determining renal function. Therefore, well-defined limits of safe WIT are lacking. Reports on kidneys harvested from non-heart-beating donors have shown favorable recovery of renal function in transplanted kidneys that sustained 45 to 271 minutes of WIT.[15–17] Despite the additional insult to these kidneys by the use of nephrotoxic immune modifiers, they have maintained good long-term renal function. Recently, authors from Cleveland[18] assessed the impact of warm ischemia on renal function, using their large database of LPNs for tumor. While agreeing that renal hilar clamping is essential for precise excision of the tumor, and other elements of the operation, the authors indicate that warm ischemia may potentially damage the kidney. However, they found that there were virtually no clinical sequelae from warm ischemia of up to 30 minutes. They also found that advancing age and pre-existing renal damage increased the risk of postoperative renal damage.

Orvieto et al[19] evaluated the upper limit for WIT beyond which irreversible renal failure will occur in a single-kidney porcine model. They concluded that renal function recovery after WIT of up to 120 minutes was not affected by the surgical approach (open versus laparoscopic). However, a prolonged WIT of 120 minutes produced significant loss in renal function and mortality in a single-kidney porcine model. Using the same model, 90 minutes of WIT allowed for complete recovery of renal function, and the authors proposed that 90 minutes of WIT may represent the maximal renal tolerance in the single-kidney porcine model.

If the warm ischemia is anticipated to be long (traditionally longer than 30 minutes), renal hypothermia is advisable before proceeding with partial nephrectomy. Experimental techniques investigated in the laboratory, such as a cooling jacket and retrograde cold saline perfusion of the pelvicaliceal system through a ureteral catheter,[20] have not been used widely clinically to date. Gill et al developed a transperitoneal technique that employs renal surface contact hypothermia with ice-slush using a laparoscopic approach. Its efficacy has been evaluated in 12 patients.[21] An Endocatch-II bag is placed around the completely mobilized and defatted kidney, and its drawstring is cinched around the intact mobilized renal hilum. The renal hilum is occluded with a Satinsky clamp. The bottom of the bag is retrieved through a 12-mm port site and cut open. Finely crushed ice-slush is rapidly introduced into the bag to surround the kidney completely, thereby achieving renal hypothermia. Pneumoperitoneum is re-established, and LPN is performed after the bag has been opened and the ice has been removed from the vicinity of the tumor. In their experience, approximately 5 minutes were required to introduce 600 to 750 ml of ice-slush around the kidney. The core renal temperature dropped to 5 to 19°C, as measured by a needle thermocouple probe. This laparoscopic technique of renal surface contact hypothermia with ice-slush replicates the method routinely used during open partial nephrectomy.[21] Further refinements in the

laparoscopic delivery system will result in more efficient and rapid introduction of ice around the kidney.

Hilar clamping

In LPN clear visualization of the tumor bed is imperative. Hilar clamping achieves a bloodless operative field and decreases renal turgor and hence enhances the achievement of a precise margin of healthy parenchyma during tumor excision, suture control of transected intrarenal blood vessels, precise identification of caliceal entry followed by water-tight suture repair, and renal parenchymal reconstruction. The controlled surgical environment provided by transient hilar clamping is advantageous for a technically superior LPN. The small completely exophytic tumor with minimal parenchymal invasion may be wedge resected without hilar clamping as it would have been performed in open surgery.[22,23]

Theoretically, the technique of hilar unclamping can create a less clear operative field and can result in uncontrolled bleeding, unidentified injuries to the collecting system, and more difficulties in identifying the correct excisional plane. Guillonneau et al[24] reported that performing LPN without clamping the vascular pedicle is associated with a significantly greater blood loss and transfusion rate.

The necessity of hilar clamping becomes clear in cases where tumor resection is difficult or complex, such as tumors that are partially exophytic with a certain depth of parenchymal invasion or are large in size. This includes tumors that are broad based in the parenchyma, completely intrarenal, abutting the collecting system, or located near the mid-portion of the kidney.

Gerber and Stockton conducted a survey to assess the trend among urologists in PN practice and found 41% of the respondents clamp the renal artery only to obtain vascular control.[25]

Many investigators have advocated clamping of the renal artery alone (rather than the whole pedicle) to allow precise excision and repair in a bloodless field, and at the same time allow continuous venous drainage to decrease venous oozing and reduce possible ischemic damage by free radicals that are produced during ischemia periods. However, isolating and dissecting the vessels in the renal hilum carries a theoretic risk of vascular injury that may necessitate total nephrectomy.

Because hilar clamping results in renal ischemia, tumor excision and renal reconstruction must be completed precisely and expeditiously.

Hemostatic aids

One of the essential elements in PN is to achieve secure renal parenchymal hemostasis. Concerns regarding hemostasis have precluded widespread use of LPN for all patients who would be candidates for open partial nephrectomy.[11,22,23]

In LPN the most commonly and securely used technique for achieving hemostasis from the significant interlobar and intralobar parenchymal vessels that are transected during LPN is precise suture ligation followed by a tight hemostatic reapproximation of the renal parenchyma (renorrhaphy) over absorbable bolsters, with the renal hilum cross-clamped, similar to open PN. The use of various hemostatic techniques and agents has been reported widely in LPN series, and is discussed briefly here.

Double loop tourniquet

This device consists of two U-loop strips of knitted tape extending from a 17 Fr plastic sheath. The device has been proposed to achieve regional vascular control by circumferential compression of the renal parenchyma during a polar PN. In describing their technique, Gill et al[26] place one double loop around the upper and one around the lower renal poles and cinch the loop around the pole containing the tumor, leaving the other one loose, thus securely entrapping the kidney and achieving a tourniquet effect. The renal artery is not occluded, hence minimizing ischemic renal damage. Additional advantages include a short WIT and maintenance of good perfusion to the uninvolved pole. Although it is effective in the smaller kidney of the experimental porcine model, such renal parenchymal tourniquets are clinically unreliable in the larger human kidney, where persistent pulsatile arterial bleeding has been noted from the parenchymal cut edge despite tourniquet deployment. Additional practical problems include the potential for premature tourniquet slippage causing significant hemorrhage, renal parenchymal fracture owing to too tight cinching of the tourniquet, and the lack of applicability for tumors in the middle part of the kidney.[26]

Cable tie

This is another tourniquet-like technique to control bleeding from the resection site. McDougall et al first reported the use of a plastic cable tie for LPN in a pig model,[3] then Cadeddu et al[27] reported its use in a clinical setting where the tumor is exposed and the cable tie is applied in a loose loop and positioned around the pole between the tumor and the renal hilum. The tie is then tightened to render the entire involved pole ischemic then the tumor is excised. A similar caveat can be made on the cable tie as for the double loop tourniquet.

Argon beam coagulator

The argon beam coagulator conducts radiofrequency current to tissue along a jet of inert, non-flammable argon gas. Argon gas has a lower ionization potential than air and consequently directs the flow of current. It may also blow away blood and other liquids on the tissue surface, enhancing visualization of the bleeding site as well as eliminating electric current dissipation in the blood. Smoke is reduced because the argon gas displaces oxygen and inhibits burning. One initial study to asses its efficacy in clinical settings comes from Postema et al,[28] who studied the blood loss, the time needed to achieve adequate hemostasis, and histologic findings after liver resection in 12 pigs using argon beam coagulation or suture ligation only, the mattress suture technique, and tissue glue application. Argon beam coagulation resulted in less tissue damage than tissue glue or mattress suturing, and the authors concluded that the argon beam coagulator is an efficient device for achieving hemostasis following partial hepatectomy in the pig and causes only a moderate tissue reaction.

In urologic literature clinical data on human PN are lacking, although its benefit as a surface coagulator can be inferred from the other parenchymal efficacy studies.

The argon beam coagulator is obviously insufficient for controlling the pulsatile arterial hemorrhage from larger intrarenal vessels.

Ultrasonic shears

Ultrasonic shears (harmonic scalpel) are a form of energy that simultaneously divides and coagulates tissue using a titanium blade vibrating at 55 000 Hz. The resulting temperature (ranging from 50 to 100°C) causes denaturing protein coagulum. In LPN this is used for tumor excision with or without vascular clamping. Harmon et al[23] evaluated its use in 15 patients undergoing LPN with small tumors (mean size 2.3 cm) without vascular clamping, and reported a mean blood loss of 368 ml and a mean operative time of 170 minutes. They confirmed the safety of this device for parenchymal resection without vascular control. Guillonneau et al[24] performed a non-randomized retrospective comparison of two techniques for LPN, that is without and with clamping the renal vessels. In group 1 (12 patients) PN was performed with ultrasonic shears and bipolar cautery without clamping the renal vessels; while in group 2 (16 patients) the renal pedicle was clamped before tumor excision. Mean renal ischemia time was 27.3 minutes (range 15 to 47 minutes) in group 2 patients. Mean laparoscopic operating time was 179.1 minutes (range 90 to 390 minutes) in group 1 compared with 121.5 minutes (range 60 to 210 minutes) in group 2 ($p = 0.004$). Mean intraoperative blood loss was significantly higher in group 1 than in group 2 (708.3 versus 270.3 ml, $p = 0.014$). Surgical margins were negative in all specimens.

Although they offer the advantage of tumor excision without vascular occlusion, and hence reduce the possibility of renal ischemic damage, the disadvantages of ultrasonic shears include tissue charring, which causes tissue to adhere to the device, creating an inexact line of parenchymal incision with poor visualization of the tumor bed. They are also inadequate as the sole hemostatic agent for controling major renal parenchymal bleeding.[29]

Water (hydro) jet dissection

Hydro-jet technology utilizes an extremely thin, high-pressure stream of water. This technology has been routinely used in industry as a cutting tool for different materials such as metal, ceramic, wood and glass. Recently, hydro-jet technology has been used for dissection and resection during open and laparoscopic surgical procedures. A high-pressure jet of water forced through a small nozzle allows selective dissection and isolation of vital structures such as blood vessels, collecting systems, and nerves. Shekarriz et al have investigated this technology during LPN in the porcine model[30] and reported a virtually bloodless field with the vessels and collecting system preserved. Moinzadeh et al[31] evaluated hydro-jet assisted LPN without renal hilar vascular control in the survival calf model. Twenty kidneys were investigated and it was found that pelvicaliceal suture repair was necessary in 5 of 10 chronic kidneys (50%), the mean hydro-jet PN time was 63 minutes (range 13 to 150 minutes), mean estimated blood loss was 174 ml (range 20 to 750 ml), and the mean volume of normal saline used for hydro-dissection was 260 ml (mean 50 to 1250 ml). No animal had a urinary leak.

Currently, no human studies for water-jet dissection in LPN have been described.

Microwave coagulation

A microwave tissue coagulator was introduced by Tabuse in 1979[32] for hepatic surgery and has subsequently been shown to coagulate vessels as large as 3 to 5 mm in diameter. This technique utilizes needle-type monopolar electrodes to apply microwave energy to the tissue surrounding the electrode. These microwaves comprise the 300–3000 MHz range of the electromagnetic spectrum and generate heat at the tip of the electrode, leading to the formation of a conical-shaped wedge of coagulated tissue.

In urology, microwave energy has been successful in prostate surgery for both benign enlargement and malignant disease. A microwave coagulator has been utilized clinically by Kagebayashi and colleagues and Naito and associates for open PN. Several other studies have reported the usefulness of this apparatus in open PN, especially in wedge resection of small renal tumors without renal pedicle clamping.[33–37] For LPN, Yoshimura et al[38] reported its use in 6 patients with small exophytic renal masses (11–25 mm in diameter) without renal pedicle clamping at a setting of 2450 MHz. The mean operating time was 186 minutes (range 131 to 239 minutes) and blood loss was less than 50 ml. Complications were mild and tolerable, and there was no significant deterioration of renal function or urinary leak. Terai et al[39] evaluated the same technique in 19 patients with small renal tumors 11 to 45 mm in diameter without hilar clamping. The mean operative time was 240 minutes with minimal blood loss in 14 patients and 100 to 400 ml loss in 4 patients. In one patient, frozen sections revealed a positive surgical margin and additional resection was performed. Postoperative complications included extended urine leakage for 14 days, arteriovenous fistula, and almost total loss of renal function, respectively, in one patient. With the median follow-up of 19 months, no patients showed local recurrence or distant metastasis by CT scan. The authors stressed the fact that the indication of this procedure should be highly selective in order to minimize serious complications secondary to unexpected collateral thermal damage to surrounding structures.

Radiofrequency coagulation

Investigators have successfully used interstitial ablative technologies (like radiofrequency ablation and cryotherapy) as definitive in situ management of select renal lesions,[40–42] but in this technique as ablated tumors are left in situ, the effectiveness of ablation in the target lesion and the cost of radiographic follow-up have created postoperative concerns, hence radiofrequency-assisted LPN emerged. Similar to microwave coagulation, radiofrequency coagulation can be used prior to partial nephrectomy to achieve energy-based tissue destruction followed by resection of the ablated tissue in a relatively bloodless field without the need for hilar clamping. In this technique radiofrequency energy is applied by electrodes placed into a grounded patient to produce an electric current. Impedance within the tissue leads to heat production, which results in temperatures sufficient to cause tissue coagulation.

Gettman et al[43] reported this technique in 10 patients with both exophytic and endophytic tumors 1.0 to 3.2 cm in diameter. The median operative time was 170 minutes and the median blood loss was 125 ml. This technique resulted in complete tissue coagulation within the treated volume, thereby facilitating intraoperative visualization, minimizing blood loss, and permitting rapid and controlled tumor resection. The renal architecture was preserved, allowing accurate diagnosis of renal cell carcinoma and angiomyolipoma in 9 and 1 cases, respectively. No perioperative complications occurred.

More recently, Urena et al[44] reported their experience with this technique in 10 patients including 9 with solid renal masses and 1 with a complex cyst. In all cases the renal hilum was dissected and the renal vessels were isolated, but none had renal vascular clamping; mean tumor size was 3.9 cm (range 2.1 to 8 cm). The mass had a peripheral location in 7 cases and a central location in 3. Mean operative time was 232 minutes (range 144 to 280 minutes) and mean blood loss was 352 ml (range 20 to 1000 ml). One patient received a blood transfusion and all tumor margins were negative. One patient had a short period of urine leakage from the lower pole calix, which was managed by ureteral stenting and Foley catheter drainage of the bladder.

Although this technique resulted in successful resection of exophytic and partial endophytic lesions in a relatively bloodless field without the need for vascular clamping, its applicability in central or deep lesions is still in question and longer follow-up for oncologic evaluation is still awaited.

Biologic tissue sealants

Biologic fibrin sealants are increasingly described in published studies for various surgical specialties,[45] and in urology these agents have been used during pyeloplasty, for ureteric repair, renal trauma, the treatment of urinary fistulae, and open and laparoscopic PN since 1979.[46–48] A recent survey of 193 members of the World Congress of Endourology revealed 68% of surgeons routinely utilized fibrin sealant to assist with hemostasis during LPN.[25]

Table 8.1 illustrates the hemostatic agents and tissue adhesives available in the United States. One example of these is the gelatin matrix thrombin sealant (FloSeal®, Baxter), approved by the Food and Drug Administration in 1999. This agent is composed of glutaraldehyde cross-linked fibers derived from bovine collagen. Its basic mechanism of action is to facilitate the last step of the clotting cascade, conversion of fibrinogen to fibrin. Furthermore, cross-linking of soluble fibrin monomers creates an insoluble fibrin clot that acts as a vessel sealant. Not dependent on the natural coagulation cascade for its efficacy, the gelatin granules (500 to 600 μm in size) swell on contact with blood, creating a composite hemostatic plug with physical bulk that mechanically controls hemorrhage.[49] Richter et al[50] and Bak et al[51]

described the use of gelatin matrix thrombin sealant in LPN. In the 16 cumulative patients in these two small series, no renal suturing was used. All tumors were somewhat superficial, with no patient undergoing pelvicaliceal repair. The median blood loss was 109 ml and 200 ml, respectively; no patient required blood transfusion and none developed postoperative hemorrhage. Another example of tissue sealant is Tisseel® fibrin sealant (Baxter Inc), a complex human plasma derivative with significant hemostatic and tissue sealant properties; this fibrin sealant includes a concentrated solution of human fibrinogen and aprotinin, which, on delivery, is mixed equally with a second component consisting of thrombin and calcium chloride. The addition of aprotinin helps to slow the natural fibrinolysis occurring at the resection site. With time, natural bioabsorption of the Tisseel will result from plasma-mediated lysis.[52]

Bovine serum albumin and glutaraldehyde tissue adhesive (BioGlue®) is another example of these sealants that have recently been introduced to urologic surgery. Glutaraldehyde exposure causes the lysine molecules of the bovine serum albumin, extracellular matrix proteins, and cell surfaces to bind to each other, creating a strong covalent bond. The reaction is spontaneous and independent of the coagulation status of the patient. The glue begins to polymerize within 20 to 30 seconds and reaches maximal strength in approximately 2 minutes, resulting in a strong implant. The degradation process takes approximately 2 years, and it is then replaced with fibrotic granulation tissue. Hidas et al[53] studied the feasibility of using BioGlue to achieve hemostasis and prevent urine leakage during open PN in 174 patients. A total of 143 patients underwent the surgery with the traditional suturing technique (suture group) and 31 patients underwent a sutureless BioGlue sealing-only procedure (BioGlue group). The use of BioGlue reduced the mean warm ischemic time by 8.8 minutes (17.2 versus 26 minutes, $p = 0.002$). The mean estimated blood loss was 45.1 ml in the BioGlue group and 111.7 ml in the suture group ($p = 0.001$). Blood transfusion was required in 1 patient (3.2%) in the BioGlue group and 24 (17%) in the suture group ($p = 0.014$). None of the patients treated with BioGlue developed urinary fistula compared with 3 (2%) in the suture group. The use of other local hemostatic agents, such as gelatin (Gelfoam, Pharmacia & Upjohn), thrombin, oxidized regenerated cellulose (Surgicel, Ethicon), and microfibrillar collagen (Avitene, Davol), has been fraught with difficulties in application, particularly in parenchymal bleeding sites without a dry surface, in difficult-to-reach locations, and by a lack of efficacy in anticoagulated patients.[50]

In renal surgery, only a few studies, none of them prospective and randomized, have tried to evaluate the

Table 8.1 Hemostatic agents and tissue adhesives available in the United States

Brand name®	Component	Manufacturer	Use
Tisseel VH, Crosseal	Fibrin sealant	Baxter	Hemostatic, tissue adhesive
FloSeal	Gelatin matrix thrombin	Baxter	Hemostatic
Thrombin-JMI	Thrombin	Jones Pharma	Hemostatic
Gelfoam	Gelatin sponge	Pharmacia & Upjohn	Hemostatic
Surgicel	Oxidized cellulose	Ethicon	Hemostatic
Actifoam	Collagen sponge	CR Bard	Hemostatic
Avitene	Collagen fleece	CR Bard	Hemostatic
NovoSeven	Recombinant factor VIIa	Novo Nordisk A/S	Hemostatic
CoSeal	Polyethylene glycol	Baxter	Tissue adhesive
Dermabond	Cyanoacrylate	Ethicon	Tissue adhesive
BioGlue	Albumin glutaraldehyde	Cryolife	Hemostatic, tissue adhesive

efficacy of tissue sealants, fibrin sealant in particular.[45–47,54] The general observation from these studies is that a relatively dry parenchymal surface is essential before application of conventional fibrin sealants and, if this can be achieved, minor venous oozing can be stopped. It is worth mentioning that a number of these investigations that addressed the effectiveness of fibrin sealant used one or more additional methods of hemostasis, such as suturing or argon beam coagulation. The disadvantages of biologic sealant technology include, in addition to its cost, allergic reaction, potential transmission of prion diseases because of its bovine derivation, and the need to mix two components and/or sequentially apply them. The risk of viral transmission with gelatin matrix thrombin sealant appears to be remote. Because they are essentially hemostatic agents, some may be ineffective for sealing collecting system entry.[49]

Fibrin sealant offers an effective adjunct for hemostasis, reinforcement of urinary tract closure, and adhesion of tissue planes,[48] but should not be viewed as a replacement for conventional sound surgical judgment or technique.

In the future, it is likely that newer potent bioadhesives may play a more significant role in obtaining renal parenchymal hemostasis.

MORBIDITY

One can make the assumption that LPN combines the advances and benefits of nephron-sparing surgery and laparoscopy to offer a decreased morbidity inherent to laparoscopy (as evident in laparoscopic radical nephrectomy compared to open), while preserving renal function, as offered by PN.

As the standard of care, when nephron-sparing surgery is contemplated, the open technique sets the standard by which LPN can be judged with respect to applicability and morbidity.

The investigators from Cleveland Clinic analyzed the complications of the initial 200 cases treated with LPN for a suspected renal tumor[55] and reported that 66 (33%) patients had a complication: 36 (18%) patients had urologic complications, the majority of which was bleeding, and 30 (15%) patients had non-urologic complications. This experienced team also reported a decreased complication rate (16%) since they began using a biologic hemostatic agent as an adjunctive measure.

Gill et al[7] compared 100 patients who underwent LPN with 100 patients who underwent open PN. The median surgical time was 3 hours vs 3.9 hours ($p < 0.001$), estimated blood loss was 125 ml vs 250 ml ($p < 0.001$), and mean WIT was 28 minutes vs 18 minutes ($p < 0.001$). The laparoscopic group required less postoperative analgesia, a shorter hospital stay, and a shorter convalescence. Intraoperative complications were higher in the laparoscopic group (5% vs 0%; $p = 0.02$), and postoperative complications were similar (9% vs 14%; $p = 0.27$). Functional outcomes were similar in the two groups: median preoperative serum creatinine (1.0 vs 1.0 mg/dl, $p < 0.52$) and postoperative serum creatinine (1.1 vs 1.2 mg/dl, $p < 0.65$). Three patients in the laparoscopic group had a positive surgical margin compared to none in the open groups (3% vs 0%, $p < 0.1$).

Table 8.2 Operative and oncologic results for LPN series with at least 20 patients

Author	Sample size	Patients with cancer (%)	Mean tumor size (cm)	OR time (Min)	Mean blood loss (ml)	Hilar control (%)	Collecting system closure (%)	Mean follow-up (months)	Complications (%)	Positive margins (%)	Recurrence	Mean hospital stay (days)
Link et al	217	66.4	2.6	186	350	75	41	12	10.6 [1]	3.2	1.4	3.1
Ramani et al	200	NS	2.9	199	247	99	71	12	33	NS	NS	2
Venkatesh et al	126	69	2.6	204	269	45	31	16	20.6	2.5	None	3
Gill et al	100	70	2.8	180	125	91	64	18	21	3	None	2
Abukora et al	78	83.3	2.2	189	233	63	30.6	17.2	29.5	1.3	None	NS
Weld et al	60	60	2.4	179	225.5	73.3	38.3	25.3	30	0	None	2.7
Rassweller	53	37	2.3	191	725	—	—	24	19	0	None	5.4
Jeschke et al	51	74.5	2	132	282	0	0	34.2	10	0	None	5.8
Guillonneau et al	28	64	2.2	158	490	57	39	7	21	0	None	4.7
Beasley et al	27	70	2.4	210	250	22	NS	NS	11	0	None	2.9
Janetschek et al	25	78.6	1.9	164	287	0	0	22.2	12	NS	None	8

NS, not stated.
(1) Only postoperative complications given.

Similarly, Beasley et al[56] retrospectively compared the result of laparoscopic PN to open PN using a tumor size-matched cohort of patients. Although the mean operative time was longer in the laparoscopic group (210 ± 76 minutes versus 144 ± 24 minutes; $p < 0.001$), the blood loss was comparable between the two groups (250 ± 250 ml vs 334 ± 343 ml; $p =$ not statistically significant). No blood transfusions were performed in either group. The hospital stay was significantly reduced after LPN compared with the open group (2.9 ± 1.5 days vs 6.4 ± 1.8 days; $p < 0.0002$), and the postoperative parenteral narcotic requirements were lower in the LPN group (mean morphine equivalent 43 ± 62 mg vs 187 ± 71 mg; $p < 0.02$). Three complications occurred in each group. With LPN, no patient had positive margins or tumor recurrence. In this Canadian study direct financial analysis demonstrated a lower total hospital cost after LPN (4839 dollars $\pm$ 1551 dollars versus 6297 dollars $\pm$ 2972 dollars; $p < 0.05$).

The operative results of large LPN series are summarized in Table 8.2. Altogether, one can conclude that LPN reduces morbidity when compared with open PN, although a solid conclusion can only be obtained with a randomized prospective comparative study with sufficient follow-up.

ONCOLOGIC RESULTS

Longitudinal studies for open PN for tumors less than 4 cm have demonstrated the efficacy and safety of this approach comparable to radical nephrectomy. Herr reported 98.5% recurrence-free and 97% metastasis-free results at 10 years' follow-up after open PN.[6] In a similar manner, Fergany et al[2] presented the 10-year follow-up of patients treated with nephron-sparing surgery at their institution, and reported cancer-specific survival rates of 88.2% at 5 years and 73% at 10 years, and this was significantly affected by tumor stage, symptoms, tumor laterality, and tumor size.

As stated in the mortality section, the open technique sets the standard by which LPN can be judged with respect to oncologic efficacy and applicability. For LPN the available series are lacking long-term oncologic data that can be utilized to assess this technique's efficacy; nevertheless, the available short-term data are encouraging.

Table 8.2 illustrates the operative and oncologic results for LPN series with at least 20 patients.[7,24,55–63] Positive surgical margins of 0 to 3% were reported, but over the available short-term follow-ups no local tumor recurrence or metastasis were observed. Overall, although the early results of LPN series are encouraging, longer follow-up will ultimately ascertain this technique's efficacy.

SUMMARY

Laparoscopic PN is a technically advanced procedure requiring laparoscopic dexterity with time-sensitive intracorporeal suturing. Duplication of established open surgical principles is important to get a substantive procedure. Currently, no consensus exists as to the best approach to LPN. Our experience with this technique is growing and the issues of renal ischemia and adequate hemostasis are evolving. Although LPN is feasible in experienced hands, only with longer follow-up can the efficacy and utility of this technique in the nephron-sparing armamentarium be demonstrated.

REFERENCES

1. Clayman R, Kavoussi L, Soper N et al. Laparoscopic nephrectomy: initial case report. J Urol 1991; 146(2): 278–82.
2. Fergany A, Hafez K, Novick A. Long-term results of nephron-sparing surgery for localized renal cell carcinoma: 10 year followup. J Urol 2000; 163(2): 442–5.
3. McDougall E, Clayman R, Chandhoke P et al. Laparoscopic partial nephrectomy in the pig model. J Urol 1993; 149(6): 1633–6.
4. Winfield H, Donovan J, Godet A et al. Laparoscopic partial nephrectomy: initial case report for benign disease. J Endourol 1993; 7(6): 521–6.
5. Finelli A, Gill I. Laparoscopic partial nephrectomy: contemporary technique and results. Urol Oncol 2004; 22(2): 139–44.
6. Herr HW. Partial nephrectomy for unilateral renal carcinoma and a normal contralateral kidney: 10-year follow-up. J Urol 1999; 161(1): 33–4.
7. Gill IS, Matin SF, Desai MM et al. Comparative analysis of laparoscopic versus open partial nephrectomy for renal tumors in 200 patients. J Urol 2003; 170(1): 64–8.
8. Winfield HN, Donovan JF, Lund GO et al. Laparoscopic partial nephrectomy: initial experience and comparison to the open surgical approach. J Urol 1995; 153(5): 1409–14.
9. Wolf JS, Seifman BD, Montie JE. Nephron-sparing surgery for suspected malignancy: open surgery compared to laparoscopy with selective use of hand assistance. J Urol 2000; 163(6): 1659–64.
10. Gill IS, Desai MM, Kaouk JH et al. Laparoscopic partial nephrectomy for renal tumor: duplicating open surgical techniques. J Urol 2002; 167(2 Pt 1): 469–77.
11. Janetschek G, Daffner P, Peschel R et al. Laparoscopic nephron-sparing surgery for small renal cell carcinoma. J Urol 1998; 159(4): 1152–5.
12. Ward JP. Determination of the optimum temperature for regional renal hypothermia during temporary renal ischemia. Br J Urol 1975; 47(1): 17–24.
13. Novick AC. Renal hypothermia: in vivo and ex vivo. Urol Clin North Am 1983; 10(4): 637–44.
14. McLaughlin GA, Heal MR, Tyrell IM. An evaluation of techniques used for production of temporary renal ischemia. Br J Urol 1978; 50(6): 371–5.
15. Nicholson ML, Metcalfe MS, White SA et al. A comparison of the results of renal transplantation from non-heart-beating, conventional cadaveric, and living donors. Kidney Int 2000; 58(6): 2585–91.
16. Kootstra G, Wijnen R, van Hooff JP et al. Twenty percent more kidneys through a non-heart beating program. Transplant Proc 1991; 23(1 Pt 2): 910–11.
17. Haisch C, Green E, Brasile L. Predictors of graft outcome in warm ischemically damaged organs. Transplant Proc 1997; 29(8): 3424–5.

18. Desai MM, Gill IS, Ramani AP et al. The impact of warm ischaemia on renal function after laparoscopic partial nephrectomy. BJU Int 2005; 95(3): 377–83.

19. Orvieto MA, Tolhurst SR, Chuang MS et al. Defining maximal renal tolerance to warm ischemia in porcine laparoscopic and open surgery model. Urology 2005; 66(5): 1111–15.

20. Landman J, Rehman J, Sundaram CP et al. Renal hypothermia achieved by retrograde intracavitary saline perfusion. J Endourol 2002; 16(7): 445–9.

21. Gill IS, Abreu SC, Desai MM et al. Laparoscopic ice slush renal hypothermia for partial nephrectomy: the initial experience. J Urol 2003; 170(1): 52–6.

22. McDougall EM, Elbahnasy AM, Clayman RV. Laparoscopic wedge resection and partial nephrectomy: the Washington University experience and review of literature. J Soc Laparoendosc Surg 1998; 2(1): 15–23.

23. Harmon WJ, Kavoussi LR, Bishoff JT. Laparoscopic nephron-sparing surgery for solid renal masses using the ultrasonic shears. Urology 2000; 56(5): 754–9.

24. Guillonneau B, Bermudez H, Gholami S et al. Laparoscopic partial nephrectomy for renal tumor single center experience comparing clamping and no clamping techniques of the renal vasculature. J Urol 2003; 169(2): 483–6.

25. Gerber GS, Stockton BR. Laparoscopic partial nephrectomy. J Endourol 2005; 19: 21–4.

26. Gill IS, Munch LC, Clayman RV et al. A new renal tourniquet for open and laparoscopic partial nephrectomy. J Urol 1995; 154(3): 1113–6.

27. Cadeddu JA, Corwin TS, Traxer O et al. Hemostatic laparoscopic partial nephrectomy: cable-tie compression. Urology 2001; 57(3): 562–6.

28. Postema RR, Plaisier PW, ten Kate FJ et al. Haemostasis after partial hepatectomy using argon beam coagulation. Br J Surg 1993; 80(12): 1563–5.

29. Jackman SV, Cadeddu JA, Chen RN et al. Utility of the harmonic scalpel for laparoscopic partial nephrectomy. J Endourol 1998; 12(5): 441–4.

30. Shekarriz H, Shekarriz B, Upadhyay J et al. Hydro-jet assisted laparoscopic partial nephrectomy: initial experience in a porcine model. J Urol 2000; 163(3): 1005–8.

31. Moinzadeh A, Hasan W, Spaliviero M et al. Water jet assisted laparoscopic partial nephrectomy without hilar clamping in the calf model. J Urol 2005; 174(1): 317–21.

32. Tabuse K. Basic knowledge of a microwave tissue coagulator and its clinical applications. J Hepatobil Pancreat Surg 1998; 5(2): 165–72.

33. Muraki J, Cord J, Addonizio JC et al. Application of microwave tissue coagulation in partial nephrectomy. Urology 1991; 37 (3): 282–7.

34. Naito S, Nakashima M, Kimoto Y et al. Application of microwave tissue coagulator in partial nephrectomy for renal cell carcinoma. J Urol 1998; 159(3): 960–2.

35. Hirao Y, Fujimoto K, Yoshii M et al. Non-ischemic nephron-sparing surgery for small renal cell carcinoma: complete tumor enucleation using a microwave tissue coagulator. Jpn J Clin Oncol 2002; 32(3): 95–102.

36. Matsui Y, Fujikawa K, Iwamura H et al. Application of the microwave tissue coagulator: is it beneficial to partial nephrectomy? Urol Int 2002; 69(1): 27–32.

37. Kageyama Y, Kihara K, Yokoyama M et al. Endoscopic mini-laparotomy partial nephrectomy for solitary renal cell carcinoma smaller than 4 cm. Jpn J Clin Oncol 2002; 32(10): 417–21.

38. Yoshimura K, Okubo K, Ichioka K et al. Laparoscopic partial nephrectomy with a microwave tissue coagulator for small renal tumor. J Urol 2001; 165(6 Pt 1): 1893–6.

39. Terai A, Ito N, Yoshimura K et al. Laparoscopic partial nephrectomy using microwave tissue coagulator for small renal tumors: usefulness and complications. Eur Urol 2004; 45(6): 744–8.

40. Gill IS, Novick AC, Meraney AM et al. Laparoscopic renal cryoablation in 32 patients. Urology 2000; 56(5): 748–53.

41. Rodriguez R, Chan DY, Bishoff JT et al. Renal ablative cryosurgery in selected patients with peripheral renal masses. Urology 2000; 55(1): 25–30.

42. Zlotta AR, Wildschutz T, Raviv G et al. Radiofrequency interstitial tumor ablation (RITA) is a possible new modality for treatment of renal cancer: ex vivo and in vivo experience. J Endourol 1997; 11(4): 251–8.

43. Gettman MT, Bishoff JT, Su LM et al. Hemostatic laparoscopic partial nephrectomy: initial experience with the radiofrequency coagulation-assisted technique. Urology 2001; 58(1): 8–11.

44. Urena R, Mendez F, Woods M et al. Laparoscopic partial nephrectomy of solid renal masses without hilar clamping using a monopolar radio frequency device. J Urol 2004; 171(3): 1054–6.

45. Shekarriz B, Stoller ML. The use of fibrin sealant in urology. J Urol 2002; 167(3): 1218–25.

46. Urlesberger H, Rauchenwald K, Henning K. Fibrin adhesives in surgery of the renal parenchyma. Eur Urol 1979; 5(4): 260–1.

47. Levinson AK, Swanson DA, Johnson DE et al. Fibrin glue for partial nephrectomy. Urology 1991; 38(4): 314–16.

48. Lapini ACM, Serni S, Stefanucci S et al. The use of fibrin sealant in nephron-sparing surgery for renal tumors. In: Schlag G, Melchior H, Wallwiener D, eds. Gynecology and Obstetrics in Urology, Vol 7. New York: Springer-Verlag, 1994: 79–81.

49. Gill IS, Ramani AP, Spaliviero M et al. Improved hemostasis during laparoscopic partial nephrectomy using gelatin matrix thrombin sealant. Urology 2005; 65(3): 463–6.

50. Richter F, Schnorr D, Deger S et al. Improvement of hemostasis in open and laparoscopically performed partial nephrectomy using a gelatin matrix thrombin tissue sealant. Urology 2003; 61(1): 73–7.

51. Bak JB, Singh A, Shekarriz B. Use of gelatin matrix tissue sealant as an effective hemostatic agent during laparoscopic partial nephrectomy. J Urol 2004; 171(2 Pt 1): 780–2.

52. Pruthi RS, Chun J, Richman M. The use of a fibrin tissue sealant during laparoscopic partial nephrectomy. BJU Int 2004; 93(6): 813–17.

53. Hidas G, Kastin A, Mullerad M et al. Sutureless nephron-sparing surgery: use of albumin glutaraldehyde tissue adhesive (BioGlue). Urology 2006; 87(4): 697–700.

54. Kram HB, Ocampo HP, Yamaguchi MP. Fibrin glue in renal and ureteral trauma. Urology 1989; 33(3): 215–18.

55. Ramani AP, Desai MM, Steinberg AP et al. Complications of laparoscopic partial nephrectomy in 200 cases. J Urol 2005; 173(1): 42–7.

56. Beasley KA, Al Omar M, Shaikh A et al. Laparoscopic versus open partial nephrectomy. Urology 2004; 64(3): 458–61.

57. Link RE, Bhayani SB, Allaf ME et al. Exploring the learning curve, pathological outcomes and perioperative morbidity of laparoscopic partial nephrectomy performed for renal mass. J Urol 2005; 173(5): 1690–4.

58. Venkatesh R, Weld K, Ames CD et al. Laparoscopic partial nephrectomy for renal masses: effect of tumor location. Urology 2006; 67(6): 1169–74.

59. Abukora F, Nambirajan T, Albqami N et al. Laparoscopic nephron-sparing surgery: evolution in a decade. Eur Urol 2005; 47(4): 488–93.

60. Weld KJ, Venkatesh R, Huang J et al. Evolution of surgical technique and patient outcomes for laparoscopic partial nephrectomy. Urology 2006; 67(3): 502–6.

61. Rassweiler JJ, Abbou C, Janetschek G et al. Laparoscopic partial nephrectomy: the European experience. Urol Clin North Am 2000; 27: 721–36.

62. Jeschke K, Peschel R, Wakonig J et al. Laparoscopic nephron-sparing surgery for renal tumors. Urology 2001; 58(5): 688–92.

63. Janetschek G, Jeschke K, Peschel R et al. Laparoscopic surgery for stage 1 renal cell carcinoma radical nephrectomy and wedge resection. Eur Urol 2000; 38(2): 131–8.

9

Nephron-sparing surgery in non-mitotic conditions – an overview

Krishna Pillai Sasidharan and Kumaresan Natarajan

INTRODUCTION

Nephron-sparing surgery is an entrenched and validated procedure in the management algorithm of renal cell carcinoma. Its deployment in non-mitotic situations, however, has not been stressed hitherto with equal emphasis. This chapter is an overview of the indications of nephron-sparing surgery in non-mitotic lesions.

There are number of factors which make nephron-sparing surgery a relatively comfortable exercise in the context of renal cell carcinoma. The focal nature of the lesion, its precise capsulation, the conspicuous interphase between the lesion and the normal renal parenchyma, and the uninfringed pararenal spaces significantly aid surgery. Many of these factors, however, are not obtained when kidneys harbor specific or non-specific inflammatory tumefactions and ill marginated lesions with extra renal ramifications.

Though there is a myriad of non-mitotic tumefactions, this chapter proposes to focus on relatively common lesions requiring nephron-sparing techniques for their excision. We have grouped such lesions as follows:

Congenital lesions

- calyceal diverticula
- moiety disease (total duplicated systems)
- simple cysts
- angiomatous malformations

Benign neoplasm

- angiomyolipoma

Acquired lesions

- renal tuberculosis
    calcifications
    cavities
- renal hydatid disease.

The detailed clinico-pathologic review of the above conditions is beyond the purview of this chapter.

CALYCEAL DIVERTICULA

A calyceal diverticulum is defined as a cystic cavity lined by transitional epithelium and connected to a minor calyx by a narrow channel. Most often they occur adjacent to an upper, or infrequently a lower pole calyx, and are categorized as type I. Infrequent type II diverticula are larger and communicate with the renal pelvis and tend to be more symptomatic.[1] An incidence of 4–5 per 1000 excretory urograms has been reported in calyceal diverticular disease, with no apparent predilection for side, sex, or age.[2] Its propensity to occur both in children and adults equally suggests a developmental etiology.[3,4] The persistence of some of the ureteral branches of the third and fourth generation at the 5 mm stage of the embryo is believed to be instrumental in the formation of a calyceal diverticulum.[5] An array of suggested acquired causes include among others the sequel of a localized cortical abscess draining into a calyx, infundibular stenosis, stone and infection mediated obstruction, and renal injury.

Hematuria, pain, and urinary infection are the principal clinical manifestations of calyceal diverticulum and they stem from stasis-related infection or true stone formation. Co-existing vesico-ureteric reflux has to be ruled out in a high percentage of children who present with urinary infection.[6]

Excretory urography with delayed films demonstrates characteristic pooling of contrast material in the diverticulum and establishes the diagnosis in most of the cases. Retrograde pyelography, computed tomography, and magnetic resonance imaging in select cases may help to configurate the diverticulum further, if necessary.

Partial nephrectomy, once a validated procedure in the management of calyceal diverticula, cannot now be reckoned as the treatment of choice. The current available treatment options include percutaneous removal of the stones and ablation of the mucosal surface, ureteroscopic expansion of the diverticular communication with removal of stones, and laparoscopic stone extraction with marsupialization of the diverticulum.[7–9]

The success of the percutaneous procedure is contingent on placement of both a safety and a working guidewire within the calyceal diverticulum. However, in some cases as illustrated here, a large stone occupying the entire diverticular space prevents the placement of the guidewires. In such cases, by exploiting regional vascular control and hypothermia, open exploration enables stone extraction, widening of the communicating channel, and obliteration of the diverticular cavity (Figures 9.1 and 9.2).

A type II diverticulum, by virtue of its larger size and direct linkage with the renal pelvis, invokes significant atrophy of the overlying renal parenchyma. Its significant size necessitates more extensive and meticulous intrarenal dissection to achieve satisfactory obliteration of its cavity. Increased renal flaccidity produced by the renal pedicle clamping and subsequent hypothermia optimizes such intrarenal dissection and aids its extirpation and marsupialization (Figures 9.3 and 9.4).

MOIETY DISEASE

Kidneys with total duplicated collecting systems possess two renal moieties and one of them may require surgical exicison due to damage sustained through either reflux or obstruction (Figure 9.5). A detailed description of duplicated collecting systems and their pathologic conditions is beyond the realm of this chapter. Some of the technicalities in excision of diseased moieties, however, require to be highlighted.

A flank approach offers excellent exposure to the moieties, principal renal vessels, and, as well as to the accessory vessels, if any, to the moieties. Excision of the diseased upper moiety, which is often dysplastic, will require identification and ligation of the upper pole vessels. Cessation of the blood supply will demarcate the diseased moiety and its interphase with the uninvolved and healthy lower moiety more precisely (Figure 9.6). In select cases, atraumatic clamping of the renal pedicle and subsequent regional hypothermia with ice-slush will aid excision of the diseased moiety under controlled conditions (Figure 9.7). The renal vessels in the pediatric age group have a propensity to develop vasospasm during dissection and this ought to be forestalled by the liberal use of topical vasodilating agents (e.g. papaverine).

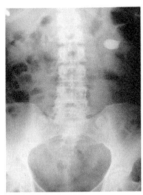
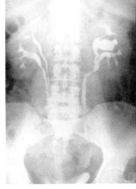

Figure 9.1 Type 1 calyceal diverticulum with stone: plain X-ray and intravenous urogram.

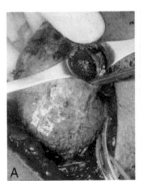
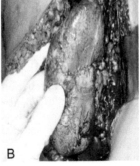

Figure 9.2 Operative photographs: (A) stone extraction and excision of the diverticulum; (B) post-repair closure of the renal parenchyma.

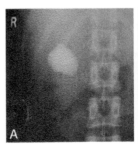
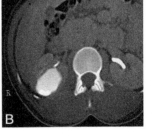

Figure 9.3 Type 2 calyceal diverticulum: (A) retrograde pyelogram (B) CT scan.

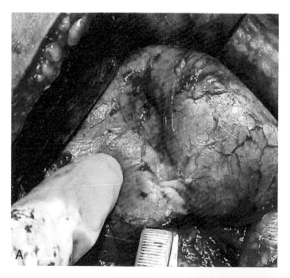
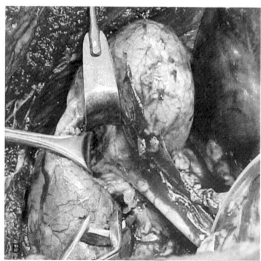

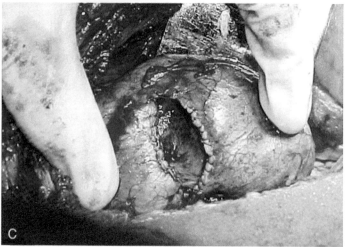

Figure 9.4 Operative photographs demonstrating (A) atrophy of the renal parenchyma overlying the diverticulum, (B) intrahilar dissection and access to the diverticulum, (C) diverticulum excision and marsupialization.

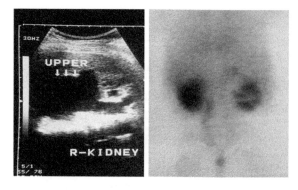

Figure 9.5 Ultrasound and radio-isotope study demonstrating right dysplastic upper moiety.

General renoprotective measures such as intraoperative use of an intravenous osmotic diuretic (e.g. mannitol) can significantly retard ischemic injuries to the retained moiety. The involved moiety is excised always with its corresponding draining ureter without stressing the blood supply to the retained sound moiety and its ureter. Laparoscopic heminephrectomy, either through a transperitoneal or a retroperitoneal route, is another surgical option increasingly employed in recent times in the realm of moiety disease. Reduced postoperative pain, earlier return of gastrointestinal function, and shorter hospital stay are the projected benefits of the laparoscopic approach and children as young as 2 to 4 months of age are not beyond this approach.[10–12]

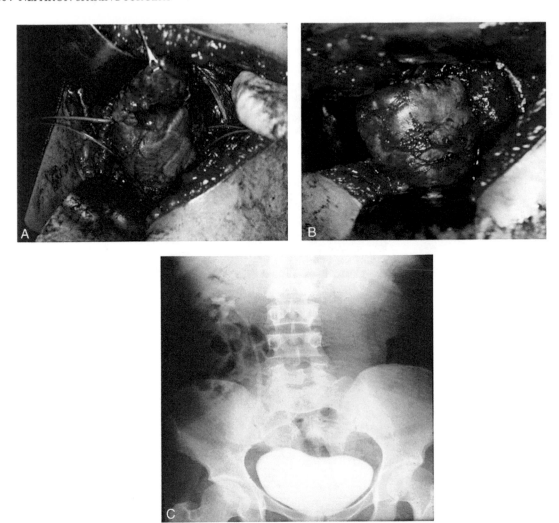

Figure 9.6 Operative photographs demonstrating (A) the excision of the diseased upper moiety, (B) closure of the parenchymal defect, (C) postoperative intravenous urogram showing preserved lower moiety.

SIMPLE CYSTS

Simple cysts invoking pain, pyelocalyceal obstruction, and hypertension may be managed by surgical unroofing of the cyst or percutaneous aspiration of the fluid. Percutaneous intracystic instillation of sclerosing agents such as glucose, iophendylate (Pantopaque), and absolute ethanol can forestall reaccumulation of fluid.[13] Cysts which defy percutaneous aspiration and sclerotherapy may be subjected to percutaneous resection or laparoscopic unroofing.[14–16]

Occasionally one encounters multiple simple cysts lying side by side within the kidney, meriting the nomenclature unilateral renal cystic disease, and this condition is presumably a discrete unilateral non-genetic entity[17] (Figure 9.8). Such a cluster of cysts disposed in a strategic renal location is amenable to nephron-sparing en bloc excision using hypothermia and regional vascular control (Figures 9.9 and 9.10). This strategy would obviate the necessity of repeated interventions.

RENAL ARTERIOVENOUS FISTULA

Renal arteriovenous (AV) fistulas are classified as congenital and acquired.[18] Congenital AV malformations are extremely rare, as indicated by sparse clinical reports as well as autopsy material. However, in recent

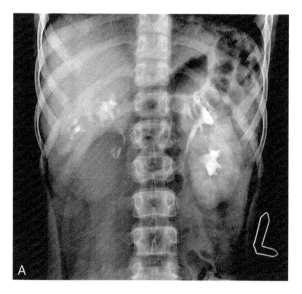
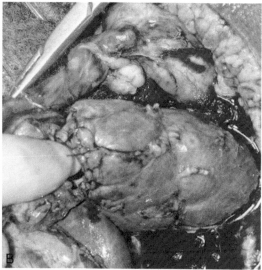

Figure 9.7 (A) Intravenous urogram demonstrating non-functioning lower moiety. (B) Operative photograph showing excision of the moiety.

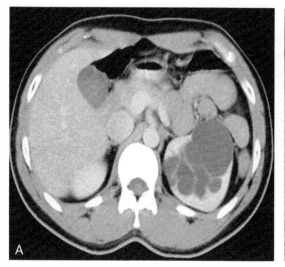
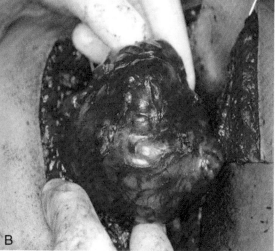

Figure 9.8 (A) CT scan demonstrating extensive unilateral cystic disease of the left kidney. (B) Operative photograph showing the cluster of cysts prior to excision.

years there has been a spurt in the incidence of acquired AV fistulas proportional to the increase in renal biopsies and other assorted percutaneous renal interventions.

The majority of renal congenital fistulas have a cirsoid configuration with multiple communications between arteries and veins, akin to congenital AV malformations in other areas of the body. The trunk and the primary divisions of the renal artery are mostly normal. The renal parenchyma also remains uninvolved, in contradistinction to acquired fistulas.[19] Spontaneous closure occurs in most of the fistulas resulting from needle biopsy of the kidney and, in a small percentage of cases, mediated through renal trauma.

Renal AV fistulas produce an array of symptoms dictated by their size and duration. Most of the symptoms are hemodynamic in character resulting from a

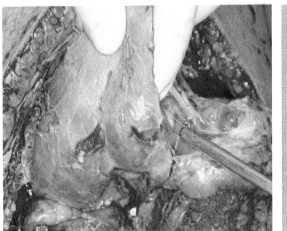
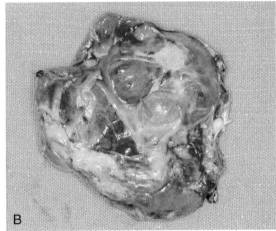

Figure 9.9 (A) Operative photograph demonstrating *en bloc* excision of the cystic conglomeration. (B) Specimen of the excised cluster of cysts.

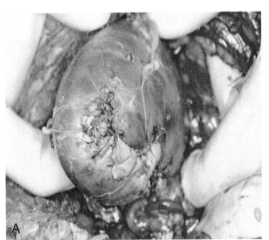
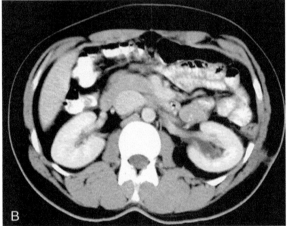

Figure 9.10 (A) The reconfigured left kidney after excision of the cysts. (B) The postoperative CT scan disclosing normal restoration of the left kidney.

high venous return and an increase in cardiac output. Long-term and persistent AV shunting may eventually lead to diminution in peripheral resistance, ventricular hypertrophy, and high-output cardiac failure.[20] Retarded perfusion of renal parenchyma distal to the fistula leads to the initiation of renin-mediated diastolic hypertension.[21]

Excretory urography may disclose diminished function focally or globally in the implicated kidney, or irregular filling defects in the pelvicalyceal system, or lesion-induced drainage impediment. These features, however, are noted in only 50% of excretory urograms. Three-dimensional

Doppler ultrasound is a reliable non-invasive method of documenting AV malformations. The lesion is always categorically diagnosed by selective renal angiography or digital subtraction angiography.

Optimal management of these benign lesions should preserve functioning renal parenchyma and obliterate symptoms and adverse hemodynamic effects associated with the abnormality. The current therapeutic options include nephrectomy, partial nephrectomy, selective embolization, and balloon catheter occlusion. Nephrectomy, once the operation most frequently resorted to, currently is exceptionally used to manage

AV malformations. AV malformations disposed at polar locations are eminently suitable for nephron-sparing curative partial nephrectomy, as in the case illustrated in Figures 9.11 and 9.12. Radiographic methods such as transluminal embolization, steel coil stenting, and balloon catheter occlusion are primarily exploited in patients with postbiopsy fistulas, where the AV connections involve small vessels and are peripherally positioned. Centrally located cirsoid AV malformations, by virtue of their diffuse distribution, preponderant communicating channels, and relatively strategic intrarenal location, pose challenging management problems. Embolization and similar radiographic methods in such cases are fraught with renal loss as well as damage to non-targeted territories.

In recent years, technologic advances in extracorporeal and microvascular surgery have permitted obliteration of difficult fistulas and subsequent vascular reconstruction in suitable cases. In-situ intrarenal disconnection of malformations is also not beyond the realm of surgical feasibility, as our illustrative case shows. Centrally located diffuse cirsoid malformations were intrarenally disconnected through a transverse division of the renal uncus under ischemic and hypothermic conditions (Figure 9.13). Renal arterial occlusion may lead to collapse of the communicating channels, making their intrarenal delineation difficult. Atraumatic clamping of the renal artery and vein and saline perfusion into the isolated vascular circuit will re-establish the AV links, rendering them easily identifiable for intrarenal disconnection.

In a few cases, as in the one illustrated here, the AV malformation extends extrarenally. Such diffuse and dense AV malformations, particularly in the hilar territory, make direct access and control of the renal artery difficult. In such cases, vascular control and renal hypothermia are effected through the transfemoral route before disconnection of the fistulas (Figure 9.14).

ANGIOMYOLIPOMA

Angiomyolipoma was originally recognized by Fischer in 1911 and designated AML by Morgan in 1951.[22] Mature adipose tissue, smooth muscle, and thick-walled vessels compose this benign neoplasm.

Its association with tuberous sclerosis syndrome (TS), an autosomal-dominant disorder characterized by mental retardation, epilepsy, and adenoma sebaceum, has been documented in about 20% of cases. Mean age at presentation in this group is 30 years, and a female to male ratio of 2 to 1 has been noted. AMLs associated with TS tend to be bilateral and multicentric, and inclined to expand more rapidly.[23] A clear female predominance and a later clinical presentation during the fifth or sixth decade are seen in patients with angiomyolipoma who do not have TS.

Flank pain, hematuria, palpable mass, anemia, and hypertension are common symptoms of AML. Massive retroperitoneal hemorrhage from AML occurs in 10% of cases and is the most bothersome complication. Currently more than 50% of AMLs are discovered

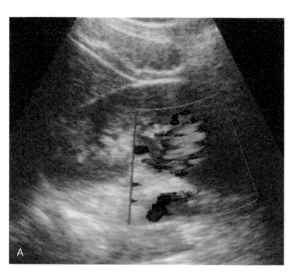
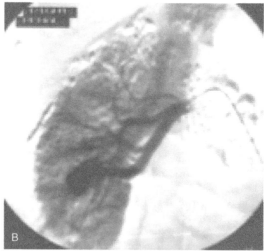

Figure 9.11 Characterization of a lower polar AV malformation by (A) color Doppler ultrasound, (B) selective angiogram.

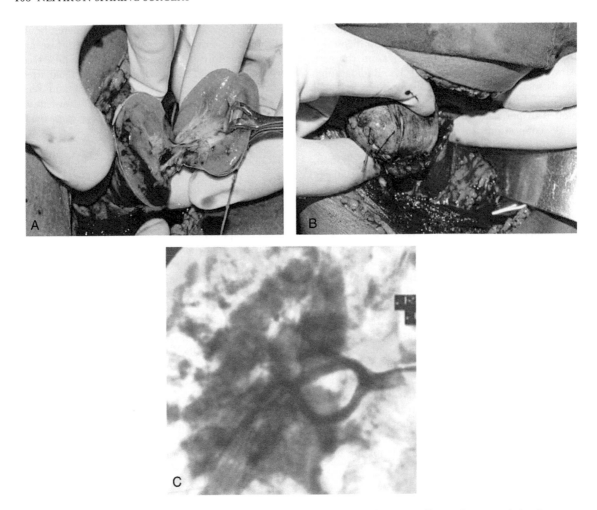

Figure 9.12 Operative photographs demonstrating (A) the excision of the AV malformation containing lower pole, (B) closure of the parenchymal defect, (C) postexcision angiogram showing the disappearance of the AV fistula. Note the absence of the feeder artery in the angiogram.

incidently due to more liberal use of abdominal cross-sectional imaging for the evaluation of non-specific complaints.

The disclosure of intralesional fat on CT scan is deemed diagnostic of AML and more or less rules out the diagnosis of renal cell carcinoma[24, 25] (Figure 9.15).

The strategies in the management of AML are dictated by the natural history and the risk of hemorrhage. There is an overwhelming consensus that AMLs of more than 4 cm in diameter tend to be symptomatic and show a greater prospensity to bleed and as such warrant intervention.[26,27] Asymptomatic smaller AMLs of 4 cm diameter or less can be subjected to periodic evaluations at 6–12 month intervals to ascertain the growth potential. AMLs in patients with TS have shown increased growth rates of approximately 20% per year, in contrast with a mean growth of 5% per year for solitary AMLs.

A nephron-sparing excision of the lesion or selective embolization of the lesion can be considered as the preferred management option in cases of AMLs requiring elective intervention. Recruited data from the literature indicate long-term success in most cases of selective embolization. Repeat embolization may be required to deal with recurrence or new lesions. Selective embolization has been found useful in the setting of life-threatening hemorrhage, bilateral disease, or pre-existing renal insufficiency.[28,29]

The preferred approach in our center in patients with AMLs is selective nephron-sparing excision of the lesion, exploiting vascular control and hypothermia. Since many AMLs contain areas of cellular atypia, it is prudent to include a rim of 0.5 cm of normal renal parenchyma to ensure radicality of excision (Figure 9.16).

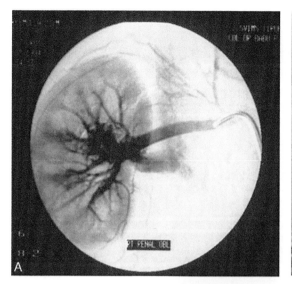
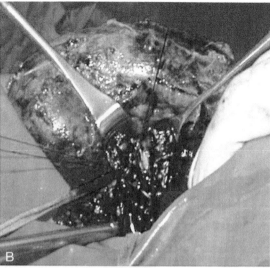
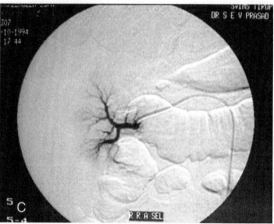

Figure 9.13 (A) Centrally located cirsoid AV malformations. (B) Intrarenal disconnection of the AV malformations through a transverse hilar nephrotomy under renal ischemia and hypothermia. (C) Postoperative selective angiogram demonstrating total disconnection of arterio-venous communications without any renal perfusion deficit.

RENAL TUBERCULOSIS

Despite the efficacy of modern chemotherapy, there are still well delineated indications for surgical interventions in renal tuberculosis. Tuberculous renal abscess cavities, granulomas, and renal calcifications remain recalcitrant due to poor regional perfusion and impeded drainage. Surgical management of such lesions improves the overall drug efficacy and ensures preservation of renal function.

Renal calcifications constitute a common and characteristic feature of tuberculosis. Although the calcifications purport to represent healed lesions, they harbor in a substantial percentage of cases viable bacilli in their matrix, and thereby promote disease recrudescence.[30] Small calcific foci may remain unchanged and can be subjected to protracted surveillance. Larger calcifications, however, expand to implicate the adjacent renal parenchyma as well as the collecting systems. Judicious excision of such calcifications is, therefore, mandatory to ensure renal preservation.[31,32]

During excision of calcifications care must be exercised to avoid collateral parenchymal damage, and vascular and calyceal infringement. Regional vascular control and hypothermia in selected cases aid tissue cleavage and detachment of calcifications from surrounding parenchyma. The density of some of the entrenched calcifications is similar to that of bone and they remain

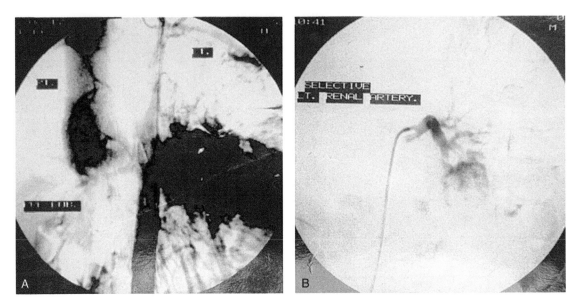

Figure 9.14 (A) Complex left renal AV malformations with significant extrarenal extension. (B) Selective angiogram demonstrating successful in-situ disconnection of the fistula. Vascular control and renal hypothermia were effected through the transfemoral route.

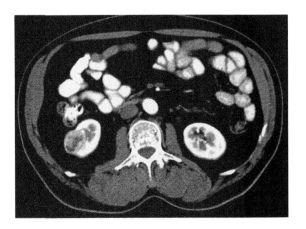

Figure 9.15 CT scan of angiomyolipoma of the right kidney demonstrating characteristic intralesional fat.

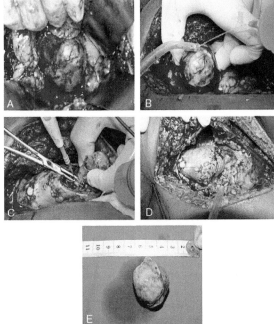

Figure 9.16 Operative photographs: (A) AML before excision, (B) and (C) process of excision, (D) closure of the parenchymal defect, (E) excised AML specimen.

refractory to intracorporeal use of energy sources such as ultrasound and lithoclast. Primary closure of the parenchymal defects resulting from excision of large and thick calcific plaques may not be possible in some instances due to tissue sclerosis as well as friability. These defects can, however, be effectively obliterated with recruitment of either perinephric fat or omentum.

Decalcification has clearly been shown to improve the renal function in many instances, as in the one illustrated in Figures 9.17 and 9.18.

Tuberculous abscess cavities can be effectively decompressed in most instances percutaneously. However, those cavities with calcific walls or containing tenacious debri and stones continue to persist promoting bacillary persistence and disease recrudescence. Most of such recalcitrant cavities are proximate to an infundibular stenosis and warrant partial nephrectomy as the best nephron-sparing option (Figures 9.19 and 9.20).

Tuberculosis-induced severe irreparable stenosis involving the upper ureter and renal pelvis warrants ureterocalycostomy to re-establish the renal drainage. This procedure mandates excision of the parenchyma overlying the lower and dependent calyx. The quantum of parenchyma to be excised is dictated by the overall thickness of the lower pole. A spatulated proximal ureter is coapted to the exposed lower calyx with appropriate sutures over an internal stent.

Surgery designed to remove tuberculosis-induced renal lesions ought to be preceded and followed by antituberculous chemotherapy to prevent urinary fistulas and systemic dissemination of tuberculosis. A combination of surgery and tuberculous chemotherapy can salvage many critically diseased kidneys, as illustrated in this chapter.

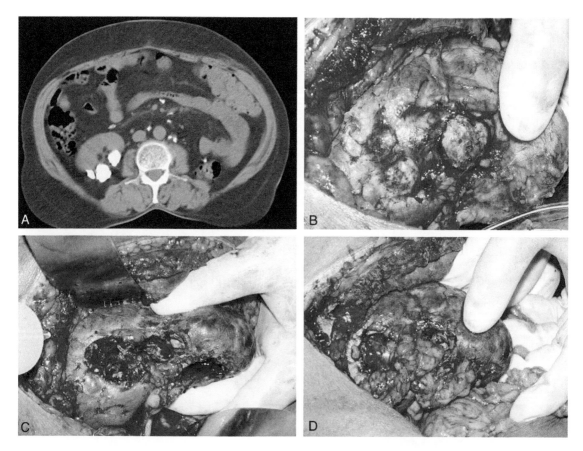

Figure 9.17 (A) Non-contrast CT scan showing large parenchymal calcifications in a patient with compromised renal function. The grossly diseased contralateral kidney was previously removed. (B) Calcifications in the process of being demarcated prior to excision. Surgery was carried out under ischemic and hypothermic conditions effected through the transfemoral route. (C) Postexcision parenchymal defects. (D) Obliteration of the parenchymal defects with mobilized pararenal fat.

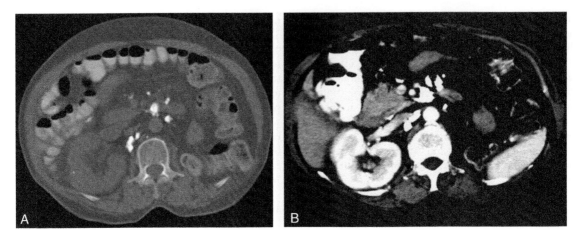

Figure 9.18 (A) Immediate postoperative non-contrast CT scan showing total clearance of renal calcifications. (B) Contrast CT 3 months later disclosing restoration of normal renal function.

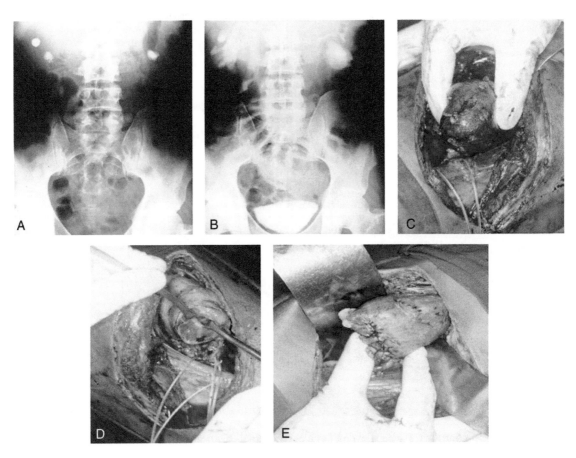

Figure 9.19 (A) Plain X-ray and (B) intravenous urogram showing stone-containing left lower polar tuberculous cavity. Operative photographs demonstrating (C) cavity prior to excision, (D) the process of excision, and (E) postexcision parenchymal closure.

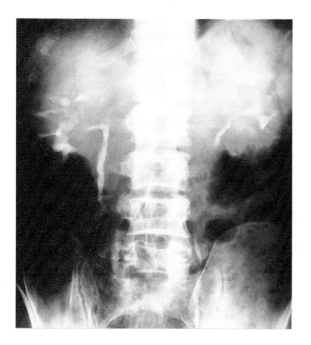

Figure 9.20 Postexcision intravenous urogram demostrating a functioning reconfigurated left kidney.

RENAL HYDATID CYSTS

The hydatid represents the larval form of *Echinococcus granulosus*. The parasite has the dog and the sheep as definitive and intermediate host, respectively. Hydatidosis is, therefore, endemic in countries with large rural sheep herding populations such as India, Africa, New Zealand, Australia, Southern Europe, and the Middle East.[33] It spares no part of the human anatomy, but renal hydatids are uncommon and account for only 2% of cases.[34]

A typical and active hydatid cyst is bestowed with three characteristic layers:

1. An outer adventitial pericyst formed by the compressed and fibrotic renal parenchyma.
2. The whitish and elastic laminated membrane (ectocyst) which is secreted by the parasite. It is chitinous and acellular in character and 1 or 2 mm in thickness.
3. The germinal layer (endocyst), a transparent and extremely thin layer, is the only living part of the hydatid cyst. It generates hydatid fluid and scolices. Each scolex represents a small inverted tapeworm head recognizable by its crown of hooklets.

Renal hydatidosis generally manifests as a solitary cyst evolving insidiously with no overt clinical manifestations for many years. It is often incidently documented on routine clinical examination, or abdominal ultrasonography. A significantly expanded cyst may cause pressure symptoms or flank pain. Rupture of the cyst into the calyceal system leads to 'hydatiduria' with the appearance of scolices and daughter cysts.

In the typical case of an uncomplicated hydatid cyst the echogenicity of the content is low, making it easily recognizable as a cyst by sonography or CT scans (Figure 9.21). The occurrence of daughter cysts is strongly indicative of hydatid cyst and they are usually readily demonstrable in both ultrasonography and CT scan. Intracystic events such as infection or hemorrhage may, however, mar the pristine imaging characteristics of hydatid cyst and make the diagnosis less straightforward. Renal hydatid disease of long duration may develop calcifications, which are usually curvilinear.[35]

Casoni's intradermal skin test and Ghedini–Weinberg's complement fixation test indicate an overall state of sensitivity to the hydatid antigen, and eosinophilia is a non-specific marker of parasitic infections. It should, however, be noted that negative serology tests do not rule out categorically hydatid disease.[36]

There are various surgical options for renal hydatid disease dictated by the size of the lesion and degree of renal involvement. These include nephrectomy, hemi-nephrectomy, and nephron-sparing excision of the cyst with its innate envelopes.

Hemi- or partial nephrectomy will ensure total extirpation of the lesion with the surrounding rim of uninvolved parenchyma. Selective excision of the cyst without infringing the pericyst also achieves a similar objective. The pericyst, a host fibrous shell, is inseparable from the renal parenchyma. This layer is, therefore, necessarily left behind when selective excision is attempted, so as to diminish the collateral parenchymal damage.

Though partial nephrectomy and selective cyst excision may be done under non-ischemic and normothermic conditions, regional vascular control and hypothermia will facilitate both procedures in renal hydatidosis (Figures 9.22 and 9.23).

Renal hydatid cysts have the propensity to induce considerable perinephric reactive changes, which obliterate the pararenal spaces and complicate dissection. Laparoscopic efforts to extirpate renal hydatids in these instances, in our experience, are fraught with frequent conversion to open surgery. Open surgery is appropriate if preoperative imaging discloses significant pararenal involvement. This approach will facilitate dissection and reduce collateral damage as well as incidence of inadvertent rupture of the cyst.

Operative spillage of cyst contents as well as leakage of the hydatid fluid lead to contamination of the

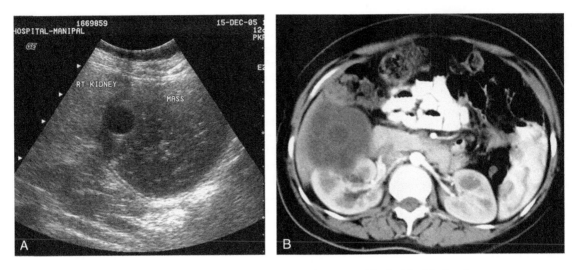

Figure 9.21 Ultrasound (A) and CT scan (B) characterize a solitary renal hydatid with daughter cysts.

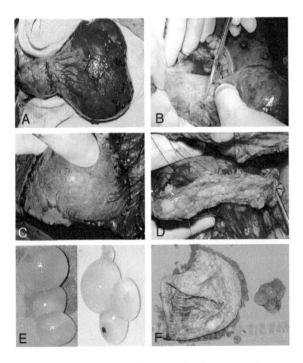

Figure 9.22 Operative photographs demonstrating (A) the hydatid cyst prior to excision, (B) the process of excision, (C) closure of the parenchymal defect, (D) reinforcement with omental free graft, (E) daughter cysts, (F) the cut-open specimen of the excised hydatid cyst.

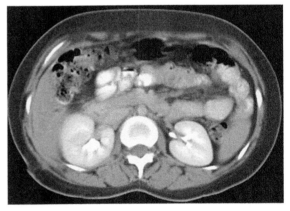

Figure 9.23 Postoperative CT scan showing normally reconfigurated and functioning right kidney.

surgical field with numerous scolices.[37] Some of these microscopic larvae will, under suitable circumstances, multiply asexually to produce new hydatid cysts. Rupture of a cyst and copious spillage of its contents may cause severe anaphylaxis. However, in recent years protracted preoperative prophylaxis with albendazole or praziquantel has significantly reduced the incidence of anaphylaxis as well as secondary echinococcosis.[38]

In selected cases percutaneous drainage of a renal hydatid cyst followed by intracystic instillation of ethanol (95%) is a validated procedure.[39] The volume of ethanol injected equals half the volume of the aspirated fluid and it is retained intracystically for 30 minutes. Percutaneous interventions are always preceded and followed by protracted courses of chemotherapy to subdue the disease activity and diminish its recurrence.

REFERENCES

1. Wulfsohn M. Pyelocaliceal diverticula. J Urol 1980; 123: 1.
2. Timmons JW Jr, Malek RS, Hattery RR et al. Caliceal diverticulam. J Urol 1975; 114: 6.
3. Mathieson AJM. Calyceal diverticulum: a case with a discussion and a review of the condition. Br J Urol 1953; 25: 147.
4. Middleton AW Jr, Pfister RC. Stone-containing pyelocaliceal diverticulum: embryogenic, anatomic, radiologic and clinical characteristics. J Urol 1974; 111: 1.
5. Lister J, Singh H. Pelvicalyceal cysts in children. J Pediatr Surg 1973; 8: 901.
6. Amar A. The clinical significance of renal caliceal diverticulum in children: relation to vesico ureteral reflux. J Urol 1975; 113: 255
7. Goldfischer ER, Stravodimos KG, Jabbour ME et al. Percutaneous removal of stone from caliceal diverticulum in patient with nephroptosis. J Endourol 1998; 12: 356.
8. Baldwin DD, Bheaghler MA, Ruckle HC et al. Ureteroscopic treatment of symptomatic caliceal diverticular calculi. Tech Urol 1998; 4: 92.
9. Hoznek A, Herard A, Ogiez N et al. Symptomatic caliceal diverticula treated with extraperitoneal laparoscopic marsupialization, fulguration and gelatin resorcinol formaldehyde glue obliteration. J Urol 1998; 160: 352.
10. Yao D, Poppas DP. A clinical series of laparoscopic nephrectomy, nephroureterectomy and heminephroureterectomy in the pediatric population. J Urol 2000; 163: 1531–5.
11. Janetschek G, Seibold J, Radmayr C et al. Laparoscopic heminephroureterectomy in pediatric patients. J Urol 1997; 158: 1928–30.
12. El-Ghoneimi A, Valla JS, Steyaert H et al. Laparoscopic renal surgery via a retroperitoneal approach in children. J Urol 1998; 160; 1138–41.
13. Holmberg G, Hietala S. Treatment of simple renal cysts by percutaneous puncture and instillation of bismuth-phosphate. Scand J Urol Nephrol 1989; 23: 207
14. Hubner W, Pfaf R, Porpaczy P et al. Renal cysts: Percutaneous resection with standard urologic instruments. J Endourol 1990; 4: 61.
15. Morgan C Jr, Rader D. Laparoscopic unroofing of a renal cyst. J Urol 1992; 148: 1835.
16. Raboy A, Hakim LS, Ferzli G et al. Extraperitoneal endoscopic surgery for benign renal cysts. In: Das S, Crawford EW, eds. Urologic Laparoscopy. Philadelphia: WB Saunders, 1994; 145–9.
17. Levine E, Huntrakoon M. Unilateral renal cystic disease. J Comput Assist Tomogr 1989; 13: 273.
18. Maldonado JE, Sheps SG, Bernatz PE et al. Renal arteriovenous fistula. Am J Med 1964; 37: 499.
19. Crummy AB Jr, Atkinson RJ, Caruthers SB: Congenital renal arteriovenous fistulas. J Urol 1965; 93: 24.
20. Messing E, Kessler R, Kavaney RB. Renal arteriovenous fistula. Urology 1976; 8: 101.
21. McAlhancy JC Jr, Black HC, Hanback LD Jr et al. Renal arteriovenous fistulas as a cause of hypertension. Am J Surg 1971; 112: 117.
22. Eble JN. Angiomyolipoma of kidney. Semin Diag Pathol 1998; 15: 21–40.
23. Neumaann HP, Schwarzkopf G, Hensk EP. Renal angiomyolipomas, cysts, and cancer in tuberous sclerosis complex. Semin Pediatr Neurol 1998; 5: 269–275.
24. Bosniak MA, Megibow AJ, Hulnick DH et al. CT diagnosis of renal angiomyolipoma: the importance of detecting small amounts of fat. AJR Am J Roentgenol 1998; 151: 497–501.
25. Jinkazi M, Tanimoto A, Narimatsu Y et al. Angiomyolipoma: imaging findings in lesions with minimal fat. Radiology 1997; 205: 497–502.
26. Oesterling JE, Fishman EK, Goldman SM et al. The management of renal angiomyolipoma. J Urol 1986; 135: 1121–4.
27. Dickinson M, Ruckle H, Beaghler M et al. Renal angiomyolipoma: optimal treatment based on size and symptoms. Clin Nephrol 1998; 49: 281–6.
28. Hamlin JA, Smith DC, Taylor FC et al. Renal angiomyolipomas: long-term effects of embolization of acute hemorrhage. Can Assoc Radiol J 1997; 48: 191–8.
29. Han YM, Kim JK, Rah BS, et al. Renal angiomyolipoma: selective arterial embolization – effectiveness and changes in angiomyogenic components in long term follow up. Radiology 1997; 204: 65–70.
30. Wong SN, Lan WY. The surgical management of non-functioning tuberculous kidneys. J Urol 1980; 124: 187.
31. Marszalak WW, Dhia A. Genito-urinary tuberculosis. S Afr Med J 1982; 62: 158.
32. Gow JG. Genito-urinary tuberculosis. In: Walsh PC, Retik AB, Vaughan ED Jr, Wein AJ, eds. Campbell's Urology, Vol 1, 7th edn. Philadelphia: WB Saunders, 1998; 807–36.
33. Gogus O, Beduk Y. Topuker Z. Renal hydatid disease. Br J Urol 1991; 68: 466–9.
34. Musacchio F, Mitchell N. Primary renal echinococcosis: a case report. Am J Trop Med Hyg 1966; 15: 168.
35. Hertz M, Zissin R, Dresnik Z et al. Echinococcus of the urinary tract: radiologic findings. Urol Rad 1984; 6: 175.
36. Matossain RM, Araj CF. Serologic evidence of the postoperative persistence of hydatid cysts in man. Hygiene 1975; 75: 333–40.
37. Mottaghian H, Saidi F. Post operative recurrence of hydatid disease. Br J Surg 1978; 65: 237–42.
38. Horton RJ. Chemotherapy of echinococcal infection in man with albendazole. Aust NZ J Surg 1989; 59: 665–9.
39. Goel MC, Agarwal MR, Misra A. Percutaneous drainage of renal hydatid cyst: early results and follow up. Br J Urol 1995; 75: 724–8.

10

Evaluation of energy sources used in nephron-sparing surgery

Ashis Chawla, Arun Chawla, and Anil Kapoor

INTRODUCTION

The increasingly available use of improved abdominal imaging modalities has led to the rise in the incidental detection of small renal tumors by almost 60%.[1] Historically, the mainstay of treatment for localized renal cell carcinoma (RCC) has been radical nephrectomy. However, nephron-sparing surgery (NSS), in particular open partial nephrectomy, has been shown to be equivalent to open radical nephrectomy in both local cancer control and overall survival, for solid renal masses less than 4 cm in size.[2-4] In addition to partial nephrectomy, needle ablative techniques are particularly useful in treatment of small renal masses, in patients where medical comorbidities may preclude major surgery. The use of energy sources in the management of renal masses has taken on an integral component in the treatment of renal masses in NSS. Firstly, the use of varying energy sources to aid in renal dissection and maximize hemostasis in laparoscopic NSS. Secondly, the adaptation of various energy sources in minimally invasive ablative techniques in the treatment of small renal masses, in patients who may not be suitable for major surgery. This chapter will explore and evaluate the use of various energy sources in these two domains in the treatment of renal masses in NSS.

ENERGY SOURCES IN LAPAROSCOPIC NSS

With the advancement of laparoscopic surgery for the management of small renal tumors, the development of new technologies for vascular control has become essential to achieving desirable surgical outcomes. With effective techniques to secure renal parenchyma hemostasis,

laparoscopic NSS may eclipse the open procedure as the standard of care for management of small renal tumors. This will allow patients to experience the benefits of decreased morbidity with laparoscopy, as well as the benefits of equivalent local cancer control; all the while, preserving the maximal amount of renal parenchyma.

The first reported laparoscopic partial nephrectomy was conducted in 1993, in a porcine model.[5] Since then laparoscopic nephron-sparing surgery (LNSS) has been incorporated in many practices, in an attempt to decrease the patient morbidity associated with the open technique. The challenge of laparoscopy lies in achieving precise tumor resection, in a relatively bloodless surgical field; all the while limiting the subsequent compromise of renal dysfunction, in timely manner.

Obtaining adequate hemostasis is essential for the advancement of laparoscopic procedures for NSS. Various techniques and strategies have been used to control hemostasis laparoscopically. A mastery of laparoscopic technical skills including suturing, clip applying, and stapling are often used to control initial bleeding. However, various energy sources such as monopolar and bipolar electrocautery, argon beam coagulators, and ultrasonic dissectors can also be used to obtain hemostasis. With a detailed knowledge of the effectiveness and limitation of each device, the laparoscopic surgeon will be able to further improve operative outcome and maximize patient safety when undertaking such complex and demanding laparoscopic procedures.

Monopolar cautery

In an attempt to incorporate open NSS into the laparoscopic arena, monopolar cautery has been widely used to obtain hemostasis in NSS. As a potential benefit, the familiarity of laparoscopic monopolar instruments – including the j-hook, laparoscopic scissors, and monopolar cautery – easily adapt from open surgery to laparoscopic NSS. Monopolar electrocautery does, however, have its limitations. Transmission of the electrocautery current through tissues of low impedance has been known to cause adjacent tissue damage. This is an important issue, especially in NSS, where preserving a maximal amount of renal parenchyma is key to desirable patient outcome. In addition, a disruption in the integrity of insulation along the monopolar electrocautery device has been demonstrated to allow for leakage of current, and adjacent tissue damage. Recognizing these limitations, several systems are in development to allow for the detection of any break in the integrity of the insulation, causing an automatic deactivation of the instrument.

Argon beam

Several other monopolar devices have been used to achieve hemostasis in NSS. The argon beam coagulator has been effectively used to control capillary bleeding in the renal parenchyma. While this monopolar instrument is effective in achieving hemostasis, it is limited in its ability to perform adequate tissue dissection. In addition, several complications have been reported, including tension pneumothorax and gas embolism.[6]

Radiofrequency monopolar devices: Tissue Link™ floating ball device

The Tissue Link device (Tissue Link Medical, Inc., Dover, NH) (Figure 10.1) is a monopolar device that uses radiofrequency energy with saline irrigation to achieve blunt dissection, hemostatic sealing, and coagulation of tumor and renal parenchyma.[7] The electrical energy is converted into heat at the tissue interface, and is facilitated with low volume saline irrigation. With a paintbrush motion, this device achieves tissue coagulation by using heat to denature the collagen matrix in both vessels and renal parenchyma. This allows for sealing of vascular structures up to 3 mm in size.[8] This device has been used to effectively perform LNSS in 10 patients, with adequate hemostasis without clamping of the renal hilar vessels.[7] The Tissue Link device limits eschar formation at the pathologic surgical margin of the specimen, allowing for accurate specimen grading and staging. Tissue Link has been shown to be a safe method for treating small peripheral renal lesions. However, deeper and more complex lesions should be approached with Tissue Link in combination with resection. In addition, Tissue Link should be minimized when used near the collecting system.

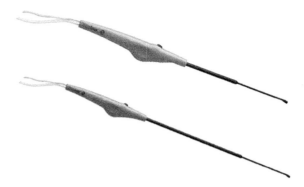

Figure 10.1 Tissue link device.

Microwave tissue coagulator

The microwave tissue coagulator has been shown to be effective in obtaining hemostasis in parenchymal bleeding in solid organs such as the spleen and liver.[9] It has also been used in open partial nephrectomy and wedge resection, without hilar clamping.[10] When used laparoscopically, the device consists of a monopolar needle type electrode, and is used in conjunction with sharp dissection of the coagulated tumor, to excise the specimen.[11] A group of 19 patients underwent LNSS using the microwave tissue coagulator. Within this series, postoperative complications included an extended urine leak, arterio-venous fistula, and impaired renal function. Additionally, a positive margin was detected in one patient. These results led the authors to suggest that the microwave tissue coagulator be used predominantly in small exophytic tumors in order to minimize serious complications secondary to unexpected collateral damage to surrounding structures.[11]

Bipolar electrocautery

Bipolar cautery has allowed for safer and more accurate dissection in NSS. With bipolar cautery, the current flow traverses between the forceps jaws only, minimizing the risk of damage to adjacent tissue and allowing for a more precise dissection. In addition to incremental sized forceps (both disposable and reusable), a bipolar radiofrequency generator and 5 mm laparoscopic Maryland style forceps (LigaSure™) are also available (Figure 10.2). The LigaSure device (Valleylab, Boulder CO, USA), uses a feedback-controlled bipolar system to deliver a precise amount of energy to vessel walls that are held in tight apposition under pressure within the jaws of the instrument. After the vessel is sealed, a cool-down phase ensues – and an audible signal identifies the end of the sealing cycle.[12] An additional advantage is minimal

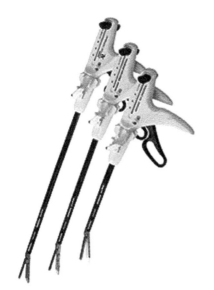

Figure 10.2 LigaSure device™.

Table 10.1 Comparison of thermal spread with varying energy devices	
Device	**Mean length of thermal spread (mm)**
Electrocautery bipolar vessel sealer[14]	2.0–3.3
Ultrasonic coagulating shears[14]	1.6–2.4

lateral spread, and thrombus formation, as well as the ability for the device to function as a tissue dissector and sealer.

The LigaSure device has been used effectively by Constant et al[12] for laparoscopic living-donor nephrectomy in 124 consecutive patients. The device proved to be highly effective for both hemostasis and dissection, with an estimated blood loss of 90 ml per case, and use of a suction device in only 32% of cases. A limiting factor in the use of the LigaSure is primarily related to its accessibility in the operative field, *vis-à-vis* laparoscopic port placement.

Ultrasound/harmonic scalpel

The harmonic scalpel is an instrument which simultaneously excises and coagulates tissue at varying frequencies. Using a frequency of 25 kHz results in dissection, whereas, a higher frequency >55 kHz will result in coagulation. The harmonic scalpel has been found to result in less transmitted thermal damage (Table 10.1), while avoiding carbonization of tissue. It has been used effectively for both retroperitoneal lymph node dissection as well as open NSS.[13,14] When used in NSS, Tomita et al[18] demonstrated that while useful for the control of renal parenchyma, larger renal vessels remained difficult to control with this instrument. Second generation harmonic instruments, including the Harmonic ACE™, may prove to be more effective at establishing hemostasis in vessels >5 mm.

Comparison of bursting pressure and thermal spread of various hemostatic devices and agents

Bursting pressure

The safety and efficacy of NSS rely largely on meticulous hemostasis in the surgical field – particularly the highly vascular renal parenchyma. Varying degrees of bursting pressure exist among the multitude of energy sources available to the laparoscopic surgeon. These pressures ultimately reflect the maximal diameter of vessels which may be safely secured and controlled via the particular energy source.

Laparoscopic titanium clips are most commonly used for mechanical coaptation of 3 to 7 mm vessels.[12] In laboratory testing these clips have been shown to have an average bursting pressure of 593 mmHg, based on an arterial vessel size of 4 mm (Table 10.1).[15–17] In comparison, polymer clips have a higher burst pressure at 854 mmHg for 4–5 mm arterial vessels.[17] Both these clips were found to be effective at pressures well above physiologic levels.

The burst pressure of bipolar electrocautery devices has been shown to be statistically higher than that achieved with ultrasonic coagulating shears/harmonic scalpel, at 601 mmHg and 205 mmHg, respectively (tested on 4 mm vessels).[17] These pressures were not statistically different for smaller vessels 2–3 mm in size.

Thermal spread

The potential complications of unrecognized thermal spread in NSS can result in significant postoperative patient morbidity. Persistent hemorrhages, development of urinary fistula, arterio-venous malformation, as well as adjacent renal parenchymal injury are all established sequelae from thermal spread. A comparison of the spread of thermal injury from ultrasonic coagulating shears and electro-thermal bipolar vessel sealing was conducted by Harold et al.[17] Using specimens stained with H&E, and examining for coagulation necrosis with light microscopy, the mean length of thermal spread in mm was identified. Coagulation necrosis ranged from 2.0 to 3.3 mm for bipolar electrocautery, whereas the harmonic scalpel ranged from 1.6 to 2.4 mm, for vessels from 2 to 7 mm in diameter. This difference was not shown to be statistically significant (Table 10.2).

ENERGY SOURCES IN MINIMALLY INVASIVE ABLATIVE TECHNIQUES

The greatest incidence in the detection of serendipitous renal masses occurs in patients above 70 years in whom associated comorbidities may preclude major surgery.[19] Needle ablative therapies are increasingly available as an alternative to extirpative nephron-sparing techniques by laparoscopic or open partial nephrectomies. The advantages of minimally invasive ablative techniques for small renal tumours include decreased morbidity, short hospital stay, reduced convalescence, preservation of renal function, and usefulness in patients with significant comorbidity. Needle-based approaches to the treatment of small renal cancers primarily involve cryoablation and radiofrequency ablation (RFA), with cryoablation being the best studied and clinically tested of the ablative procedures.

Cryotherapy

Tissue–ice interactions

Freezing temperatures in medical practice can be used for both the preservation and destruction of tissues. Once exposed to freezing temperatures, both acute and delayed histologic effects are seen in the affected tissues.[20] Acute tissue injury results from ice formation in the extracellular space, increasing the osmotic concentration and ultimately resulting in a net movement of water out of the cells to the extracellular space. This eventually leads to protein denaturation and the mechanical disruption of the cell membrane due to ice deposition in the extracellular space.[21] Endothelial injury caused during the acute phase results in microvascular thrombosis and delayed cell death because of diminished tissue perfusion.[22] This delayed effect can be demonstrated within a few hours to days after cryoablation. Tissue destruction is achieved by both the freeze and thaw processes. Double freezing when compared with a single-freeze approach, has been shown to produce greater necrosis in an animal model.[23]

Tissue freezing and ice ball monitoring endpoints

Cryotherapy aims at decreasing the temperature in the target tissue to below the level that causes complete tissue necrosis. Chosy et al[24] and Campbell et al[25] substantiated that complete necrosis in renal tissue can be attained by exposing the target tissue to less than 19.4°C.[24,25] Temperatures of −40°C are used to achieve ablation effects for renal tumors. Thermocouples placed at the tumor margin help in measuring the temperature endpoint of −40°C; alternatively, ultrasound can be used to verify extension of the ice ball 1 cm beyond the margin of the tumor. The most commonly used cryogens include liquid nitrogen and argon.

Technical considerations

The various steps involved in the cryoablation process of a renal tumor are:

- real-time imaging of the tumor
- planning for the depth and angle of entry of the cryoprobe in the tumor

Table 10.2 Comparison of bursting pressure with varying hemostatic devices		
	Bursting pressure (mm/Hg)/ arterial size (mm)	Special instruments
Titanium clips[11,12,14]	593 (4 mm)	Clip appliers (reusable/single use)
Polymer clip[14]	854 (4 mm)	Clip applier (reusable)
Electrocautery[15]	230	Reusable
Harmonic scalpel[14]	205 (4 mm)	Specific generator – single use
Bipolar vessel sealer[14]	601 (4 mm)	Standard generator – re-useable

- needle biopsy of the tumor
- cryoprobe insertion into the tumor
- creation of a cryolesion about 1 cm larger than the tumor
- hemostasis after the procedure.

Renal cryoablation can be achieved by open surgery, the laparoscopic approach, or the percutaneous technique (Figures 10.3 and 10.4).

Laparoscopic cryoablation

The laparoscopic procedure consists of proper exposure of the tumor by careful dissection of adjacent structures away from the tumor, resection of overlying perinephric fat for biopsy, precise planning for probe insertion, and ice ball monitoring under visual and ultrasound control. Anterior and anteromedial tumors are approached

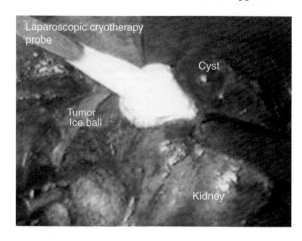

Figure 10.3 Laparoscopic cryoablation.

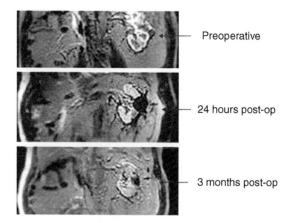

Figure 10.4 Cryoablation: pre-operative and post-operative CT imaging.

through the transperitoneal approach, while posterior and posterolateral tumors may be accessed retroperito-neoscopically.

Cryoprobes are available in various sizes of 1.5 to 8 mm diameter, but the commonly used cryoprobes are of 3.8 and 4.8 mm diameter. Follow-up imaging may include MRI of the cryolesion performed at 1, 3, 6, 12, 18, and 24 months, and annually thereafter. Abnormal findings on MRI during the follow-up warrant image guided biopsy to rule out the presence of viable tumor.

Percutaneous cryoablation

Percutaneous cryoablation is performed for posterior tumors to avoid the risk of visceral injuries. This procedure is currently performed with the use of CT scans or the newly introduced open gantry MRI scan. MRI offers the advantage of three-dimensional pictures of better definition and great clarity. Percutaneous cryoablation can be performed under mild sedation or general anesthesia. Patients with multiple tumors occurring over their lifetime, as in Von Hippel–Lindau disease, are particularly suitable for percutaneous cryoablation. Percutaneous ablation may be done under laparoscopic guidance as well.

Oncologic outcomes with cryoablation

Gill reported a series of 115 patients treated with renal cryoablation in which mean tumor diameter was 2.3 cm, mean cryoablation time was 19.5 minutes, and mean blood loss was 87 ml. Of these patients, 56 completed a follow-up of 3 years. The cryolesion size reduced by 75% at the end of 3 years,[26] and only 2 of the patients were found to have residual tumor. Cestari et al, in their series of 37 patients treated by laparoscopic cryoablation, reported no recurrence at the mean follow-up of 20.5 months.[27] Shingleton and Sewell, in their series of 22 tumors treated by percutaneous renal tumor ablation under MRI guidance, demonstrated no evidence of recurrence or new tumor development during 14 months of follow-up.[28] Bachman et al reported retroperitoneoscopic cryoablation with multiple ultrathin probes of 1.5 mm diameter. They had no residual tumor or recurrence after a mean follow-up of 13.6 months in their series and contended that the ultrathin probes have the potential to decrease hemorrhagic complications associated with the cryoablation.[29]

Complications with cryoablation

Gill et al, in their cohort of 56 patients followed up to 3 years, reported no significant effect of cryoablation on renal function.[30] In an experimental animal study,

Campbell et al reported one case of uretero-pelvic junction obstruction.[25] Pain and paresthesia at the site of probe insertion are the most commonly encountered side-effects of cryoablation and usually subside with expectant management. Other complications such as perirenal hematoma, renal fracture, and obstruction at the uretero-pelvic junction occur rarely. Renal fracture can be prevented by careful planning of perpendicular probe entry into the tumor and maintaining this position during the procedure.[31]

Renal cryoablation is both a technically feasible and safe minimally invasive procedure for the destruction of both solid and complex renal lesions. Existing short-term and intermediate-term results support the use of cryoablation for small localized renal tumors. Cryoablation can achieve excellent cancer related outcomes with follow-up of up to 110 months. Although cancer-specific outcomes are excellent, scrupulous long-term follow-up is required for determining the long-term role of cryotherapy in the treatment algorithm for small renal tumors.[31]

Radiofrequency ablation

Radiofrquency ablation (RFA) for small renal tumors was first described by Zlotta et al in 1997[32] and has now become a commonly applied percutaneous ablative technique for renal tumors.

Mechanism of action

RFA primarily results in thermal tissue damage by delivering heat (temperature >50°C) to target tissue. High-frequency alternating current flows from the needle electrode to the target tissue resulting in ionic and molecular changes, denaturation of cellular proteins, melting of membrane lipids, and eventually disruption of the cell membrane. Temperatures of 50°C produce tissue changes in 5 minutes, whereas temperatures greater than 60°C produce immediate effects. Higher temperatures (>105°C) result in boiling and vaporization of the tissue, resulting in gas formation, which can in fact interfere with further RFA. Histologically, the acute phase consists of coagulative necrosis, epithelial edema, and marked stromal changes in RF lesions. In the chronic phase, healing occurs by tissue fibrosis in the radiolesion.

To achieve the desired effect on larger tumors, the efficacy of the RFA can be enhanced by various modifications. In dry RFA, the increase in the tissue impedance caused by the increase in the tissue temperature around the probe helps in arresting further expansion of the lesion. In wet RFA, centrifugal dissipation of energy is facilitated by the use of saline irrigation which enhances the conductivity of the tissue and thus results

in a larger size RF lesion.[34] Temperature-sensing thermocouples can be used to assess the efficacy of RFA. Bipolar RFA results in a more precise lesion without the risk of accidental associated thermal injuries to other organs as compared to the monopolar RFA.[35] Various shapes of RFA devices exist, such as the umbrella mechanism which disseminates energy at various points to produce a larger ablation size.

The location of the tumor also influences the outcome of RFA. Peripheral, exophytic tumors draped by relatively avascular perinephric fat are more effectively ablated by RFA than centrally placed endophytic tumors. In these centrally positioned tumors, the surrounding vascular parenchyma results in dissipation of heat energy away from the tumor, decreasing the effective tumor ablation.[36]

Radiofrequency ablation technology

Three different types of RF energy-generating systems are available in the United States for ablation of renal tumors:

- Starburst model
- Cool-tip system
- LeVeen model.

Starburst model
The RITA model 1500X generator is a temperature based system that produces energy up to 250 W and is supplied by RITA Medical Systems. Different varieties of probes including an MRI-compatible construct (Starburst) are available for use. RF probes of 14 G with a 9-array configuration and lengths of 12 and 25 cm are available for percutaneous and laparoscopic use.

Cool-tip system
This system is a 200 W energy-based model and is marketed by Valley Lab. Single electrodes of 10-, 15-, 20-, and 25-cm length with a tip exposure of 1, 2, and 3 cm are available. Cluster electrodes are also available in 10-, 15-, and 20-cm lengths with a tip exposure of 2 to 5 cm. The 17 G electrode is cooled with cold water internally, thus reducing the temperature at the probe tip and hence decreasing the impedance in the surrounding tissue to achieve a larger RF lesion.

LeVeen model
This model comes with the LeVeen electrode of the multitine configuration. The LeVeen needle electrode has an umbrella-shaped array with a diameter of 2, 3, 3.5, 4, or 5 cm and tines separated by 1 cm (Figure 10.5). Cannula lengths of 12, 15, and 25 cm and different

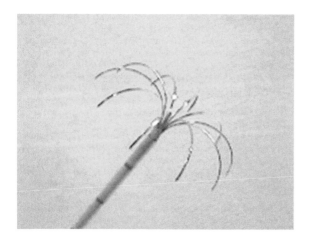

Figure 10.5 LeVeen™ needle electrode.

diameters of the LeVeen CoAccess electrode are available. The new 17 G SuperSlim LeVeen needle is available in 15- and 25-cm lengths with a 2- or 3-cm array diameter. This RFA model manufactured by Boston Scientific is an impedance-based device that provides energy up to 200 W.

Technique

Renal tumor ablation with RFA can be achieved by minimally invasive approaches including laparoscopic and percutaneous techniques. In both the techniques, the sequence of events for RFA consists of:

- image-guided localization of the tumor
- needle biopsy of the tumor
- RFA probe insertion
- ablation 0.5 to 1 cm beyond the tumor margins
- biopsy and contrast scans to check for any viable tumor.

Posterior or laterally placed tumors may be ablated percutaneously whereas anteriorly situated tumors are ablated laparoscopically. Image-guided RFA probe insertion is done via ultrasound, CT, and MRI. The size of the RF lesion depends on the ablation time, amount of energy delivered, the surface area of the electrodes, and the tissue impedance.[35] Once the RFA probe is activated, the generation of microbubbles and the hyperechoic peripheral rim of the RF lesion limit the use of ultrasound as real-time imaging. Intravenous contrast injection at the end of the procedure with the probe in position helps in assessing the enhancement on CT or MRI. Lack of enhancement of the RFA lesion after contrast injection is used as an indication of tissue ablation.

However, inflammatory changes at the periphery may present as contrast enhancement on CT or MRI if performed immediately after the procedure.

Laparoscopic RFA

In this technique, transperitoneal laparoscopic mobilization of structures overlying the tumor is conducted. The RFA probe is introduced perpendicular to the surface of the tumor. Laparoscopic ultrasound is used to locate endophytic renal tumors. The ablative tines are adjusted to create an ablation zone of 0.5 to 1 cm beyond the largest tumor diameter on cross-sectional imaging. Once the target temperature is achieved, a cool-down period of half to one minute ensues, followed by a second ablative cycle. A tumor biopsy is done at the conclusion of the procedure and extra cycles of ablation time are used whenever the RFA effect appears incomplete on visual, radiographic, or biopsy findings.

The first report on laparoscopic RFA was described by Yohannes et al for a 2-cm renal tumor ablated through the retroperitoneoscopic approach in a patient of renal insufficiency.[35] Jacomides et al, in their series of laparoscopic RFA ablation of 17 tumors, reported no recurrence or metastasis after a follow-up of 9.8 months.[37] Matsumoto et al reported 64 cases of RFA and reported only 2 failures, which were retreated by RFA.[38]

Percutaneous RFA

After general anesthesia, the patient is placed in the prone or decubitus position depending upon the tumor location in the CT or open MRI gantry. The RFA probe is passed percutaneously to create an ablation of 0.5 to 1 cm beyond the margin after preliminary biopsy of the tumor. Tract ablation is performed at the end of procedure to reduce bleeding complications.

In the initial series reported by Pavlovich et al[39] and Pautler et al[40] on the percutaneous RFA of 19 small renal masses (mean diameter of 2.5 cm), 23% had residual enhancement. At the end of 24 months' follow-up, the recurrence rate was 40%. Gervais et al treated 34 patients with 42 renal tumors using single and cluster cooled-tip electrodes under CT or ultrasound guidance with no metastasis after a maximum follow-up of 42.6 months.[41] McGovern et al, in their study of RFA in 55 patients, reported 1 ureteric stricture and 2 significant perinephric hematomas.[42]

Patients treated by RFA are followed by contrast-enhanced CT or MRI at regular intervals of 6 weeks, 3 months, 6 months, and every 6 months thereafter. Recurrence is defined as any new enhancement (>10 HU) after a non-enhancing 6-week scan. Residual and recurring tumors can be retreated by RFA or surgery.

Morbidity with RFA

Most commonly associated complications with RFA include pain and paresthesias at the site of probe insertion. Other complications include perinephric hematoma, tract bleeding, and thermal injury to the liver. Ureteral-pelvic junction (UPJ) obstruction and tumor seeding of the percutaneous tract may occur. The incidence of tract bleeding and tumor seeding can be minimized by coagulating the percutaneous channel during RFA probe withdrawal. In order to reduce complications, RFA is offered to tumors situated >1 cm away from the UPJ, not abutting it, and 1 cm from segmental renal vessels.[31]

When comparing renal RFA to cryotherapy in a porcine model, Brashears et al concluded that cryoablation was a safer option in central renal tumors as it did not cause bleeding, urinary fistula, or other significant complications but did produce reproducible areas of necrosis.[43] Similar observations have been reported by Sung et al.[44]

Renal RFA is a safe and effective treatment modality for small renal masses situated away from the collecting system and renal hilum, in elderly patients with comorbid states, and in patients not suitable for extirpative techniques by laparoscopic or open surgery. Evolution of probes of the multitine configuration facilitates the ablation of larger lesions, and the use of high-powered generators can minimize the need for retreatment. Early results in RFA series are promising, with combined local and distant disease control in 96 to 98% at 1 year;[45,46] however, longer follow-up is needed to establish its efficacy in the treatment of small renal tumors.

CONCLUSION

The use of energy sources in the area of NSS has become an increasingly important field of study over the last decade. The emerging roles of both laparoscopic NSS and minimally invasive needle ablative therapies in the treatment of renal masses have established them as effective treatments of renal cell carcinoma. It behooves the well informed urologist to foster an understanding of the various energy modalities used in NSS, in order to maximize treatment options and patient outcomes.

REFERENCES

1. Luciani LG, Cestari R, Tallargio C. Incidental renal cell carcinoma – age and stage characterization and clinical implications: study of 1092 patients (1982–1997). Urology 2000; 56: 58–62.
2. Licht MR, Novick AC. Nephron sparing surgery for renal cell carcinoma. J Urol 1993; 145: 1.
3. Campbell SC, Novick AC, Streem SB et al. Complications of nephron sparing surgery for renal tumors. J Urol 1994; 154: 1177.
4. Licht MR, Novick AC, Goormastic M. Nephron sparing surgery in incidental versus suspected renal cell carcinoma. J Urol 1994; 152: 39.
5. McDougall EM, Clayman RV, Chandhoke PS et al. Laparoscopic partial nephrectomy in the pig model. J Urol 1993; 149: 1633.
6. Shanberg AM, Zagnoev M, Clougherty TP. Tension pneumothorax caused by the argon beam coagulator during laparoscopic partial nephrectomy.
7. Urena R, Mendez F, Woods M et al. Laparoscopic partial nephrectomy of solid renal masses without hilar clamping using a monopolar radio frequency device. J Urol 2004; 171: 1054.
8. Espat NJ, Helton WS. TissueLink floating ball assisted colorectal hepatic metastasectomy. Department of Surgery, University of Illinois. Available at www.tissuelink.com.
9. Tabuse K. Basic knowledge of a microwave tissue coagulator and its clinical applications. J Hepatobil Pancreat Surg 1998; 5: 165.
10. Matsui Y, Fujikawa K, Hiroshi I et al. Application of microwave tissue coagulator; is it beneficial to partial nephrectomy? Urol Int 2002; 69: 27.
11. Terai A, Noriyuki I, Yoshimura K et al. Laparoscopic partial nephrectomy using microwave tissue coagulator for small renal tumors: usefulness and complications. Eur Urol 2004; 45: 744.
12. Constant DL, Florman SS, Mendez F et al. Use of the LigaSure vessel sealing device in the laparoscopic living-donor nephrectomy. Transplantation 2004; 78: 1661.
13. Janetscheck G, Hobisch A, Peschel R et al. Laparoscopic retroperitoneal lymph node dissection. Urology 2000; 55: 136.
14. Tomita Y, Koike H, Takahashi K et al. Use of the harmonic scalpel for nephron-sparing surgery in renal cell carcinoma. J Urol 1998; 159: 2063.
15. Kennedy J, Stranahan PL, Taylor KD et al. High-burst-strength, feedback-controlled bipolar vessel sealing. Surg Endosc 1998; 12: 876.
16. Godje O, Koukal C, Hannekum A. Electrical vessel sealing with the LigaSure system – first results in saphenous vein harvesting. Thorac Cardiovasc Surg 2000; 48(Supple 1): 8.
17. Harold KL, Pollinger BD, Matthews KW et al. Comparison of ultrasonic energy, bipolar thermal energy, and vascular clips for hemostasis of small-, medium-, and large-sized arteries. Surg Endoscop 2003; 17: 1228.
18. Klingler CH, Remzi M, Marberger M et al. Hemostasis in laparoscopy. Eur Urol 2006; 50: 948.
19. Chow WH, Devassa SS, Warren JL et al. Rising incidence of renal cell cancer in United States. JAMA 1999; 281: 1628–31.
20. Baust J, Gage AA, Ma H et al. Minimally invasive cryosurgery – technological advances. Cryobiology 1997; 34: 373–84.
21. Acker JP, Larese A, Yang H et al. Intracellular ice formation is affected by cell interactions. Cryobiology 1997; 34: 42–69.
22. Gill IS, Novick AC. Renal cryosurgery. Urology 1999; 54: 215–9.
23. Wooolley ML, Schulsinger DA, Durand DB et al. Effect of freezing parameters on tissue destruction following renal cryoablation. J Endourol 2002; 16: 519–22.
24. Chosy SG, Nakada SY, Lee FT et al. Monitoring renal cryosurgery; predictors of tissue necrosis in swine. J Urol 1998; 159: 1370–4.
25. Campbell SC, Krishnamurthi V, Chow G et al. Renal cryosurgery: experimental evaluation of treatment parameters. Urology 1998; 52: 29–33.
26. Kaouk JH, Aron M, Rewcastle JC et al. Cryotherapy: clinical end points and their experimental foundations. Urology 2006; 68(Suppl): 38–44.
27. Cestari A, Guazzoni G, Dellacqua V et al. Laparoscopic cryoablation of solid renal masses: intermediate term follow-up. J Urol 2004; 172: 874–7.
28. Shingleton WB, Sewell PE. Percutaneous renal tumour cryoablation with MRI guidance. J Urol 2001; 165: 773–6.

29. Bachman A, Sulser T, Jayet C et al. Retro-peritoneoscopy assisted cryoablation of renal tumours using multiple 1.5 mm ultrathin cryoprobes: a preliminary report. Eur Urol 2005; 47: 474–9.

30. Gill IS, Remer EM, Hasan WA et al. Renal cryoablation: outcome at 3 years. J Urol 2005; 173: 1903–7.

31. Jonson DB, Solomon SB, Liming SU et al. Defining the complications of cryoablation and radiofrequency ablation of small renal tumours: a multi-institutional study. J Urol 2002; 170: 619–22.

32. Hegarty NJ, Gill IS, Desai MM et al. Probe ablative nephron-sparing surgery: cryoablation versus radiofrequency ablation. J Urol 2006; 68(Suppl): 7–13.

33. Zlotta AR, Wildschutz T, Raviv G et al. Radiofrequency interstitial tumour ablation (RITA) is a possible new modality for treatment of renal cancer – ex vivo and in vivo experience. J Endourol 1997; 11: 251–8.

34. Hoey MF, Mulier PM, Leveillee RJ et al. Transurethral prostate ablation with saline electrode allows controlled production of larger lesions than conventional methods. J Endourol 1997; 11: 279–84.

35. Zagoria RJ, Hawkins AD, Clark PE et al. Percutaneous CT guided radiofrequency ablation or renal neoplasms; factors influencing success. Am J Roentgenol 2004; 183: 201–7.

36. Yohannes P, Pinto P, Roatariu P et al. Retroperitoneoscopic ablation of solid renal mass. J Endourol 2001; 15: 845–9.

37. Jacomides L, Ogan K, Watumull L et al. Laparoscopic application of radiofrequency energy enables in situ renal tumour ablation and partial nephrectomy. J Urol 2003; 169: 49–53.

38. Matsumoto ED, Watumull L, Johnson DB et al. The radiographic evolution of radiofrequency ablated tumours. J Urol 2004; 172: 45–8.

39. Pavlovich CP, Wood BJ, Choyke PL et al. Percutaneous radiofrequency ablation of small renal neoplasms; initial clinical series. J Urol 2001; 165: 157 (abstract 647).

40. Pautler SE, Pavlovich CP, Choyke PL et al. Percutaneous radiofrquency ablation of renal tumours: 1-year follow-up. J Urol 2002; 167: 167 (abstract 772).

41. Gervais DA, McGovern FJ, Wood BJ et al. Radiofrequency ablation of renal cell carcinoma: early clinical experience. Radiology 2000; 217: 665–72.

42. McGovern FJ, McDougal S, Gervais DA et al. Percutaneous radiofrequency ablation of human renal cell carcinoma. J Urol 2003; 169: 2 (abstract 7).

43. Brashears JH III, Raj GV, Crisci A et al. Renal cryoablation and radio-frequency ablation: an evaluation of worst case scenarios in a porcine model. J Urol 2005; 173: 2160–5.

44. Sung GT, Gill IS, Hsu TH et al. Effect of intentional cryo-injury to the renal collecting system. J Urol 2003; 170: 619–22.

45. Deane LA, Clayman RV. Review of minimally invasive renal therapies: needle based and extracorporeal. J Urol 2006; 68(Suppl 1A): 26–37.

46. Matsumoto ED, Johnson DB, Ogan K et al. Short term efficacy of temperature-based radiofrequency ablation of small renal tumours: intermediate results. Urology 2005; 65: 877–81.

11

Controversies in nephron-sparing surgery

Kumaresan Natarajan and Krishna Pillai Sasidharan

INTRODUCTION

Robson, through his landmark articles published in 1963 and 1969, very emphatically demonstrated improved survival in renal cell carcinoma after radical nephrectomy.[1,2] Since then radical nephrectomy has been the gold standard treatment for renal cell carcinoma. In the following years, nephron-sparing surgery has emerged as a logical treatment in cases of absolute or imperative indications covering clinical situations such as renal cell carcinoma in solitary kidney, bilateral tumors, and von Hippel–Lindau disease, etc. In these situations nephron-sparing surgery would forestall the morbidity of an anephric state and dependence on dialysis or renal transplantation for survival.

A further well delineated indication for nephron-sparing surgery includes renal cell carcinoma in patients with impaired contralateral renal function or at risk for future compromise. Such relative indications encompass benign conditions like nephrolithiasis, recurrent infections, vesicoureteric reflux with or without renal scarring, and obstruction or vascular insufficiency in the contralateral kidney. In most of these patients, nephron-sparing surgery is offered to circumvent future renal insufficiency or dialysis.

The relative indication can also be expanded to include individuals who have a risk of future renal compromise stemming from medical diseases such as diabetes and hypertension. In select individuals with tumor multi-focality, particularly those with a papillary variant, and in patients with underlying genetic syndromes predisposing to multifocality (e.g. von Hippel–Lindau disease), nephron-sparing surgery can be construed as a prudent treatment option.

The principal controversy regarding nephron-sparing surgery centers round its use in localized renal cell carcinoma with a normal contralateral kidney.[3,4] In recent times there are convincing reports that in single, small (less than 4 cm) kidney tumors with a normal contralateral kidney, nephron-sparing surgery is as safe and effective as radical nephrectomy.[3,4] The reported incidence of 10 to 20% tumor multicentricity has generated some concern about the chances of surgical failure after nephron-sparing effort.[5-7] Despite these tentative reservations, elective partial nephrectomy in the last decade has expanded its role in the management protocol of renal cell carcinoma. More liberal use of cross-sectional imaging in recent times for the routine evaluation of multiple abdominal disorders has significantly escalated the number of incidentally discovered small asymptomatic tumors in young and relatively healthy individuals. This ongoing scenario continues to provide the appropriate impetus for the migration of elective partial nephrectomy into the management algorithm of renal cell carcinoma.

Despite the relatively well circumscribed indications for nephron-sparing surgery in the current management of renal cell carcinoma, it is not entirely bereft of controversies. Most of the current controversies that have emerged are in relation to issues connected to the performance of nephron-sparing surgery. The issues such as the upper limit of the tumor size for elective nephron-sparing surgery, methods of excision, optimal surgical margin, impact of tumor location, and multifocality have generated divergent view points. This chapter proposes to review the controversies surrounding the above strategic issues in relation to nephron-sparing surgery.

TUMOR SIZE

Although radical nephrectomy continues to be reckoned the accepted treatment for unilateral renal cell carcinoma with a normal contralateral kidney, recruited data categorically delineate a select group of patients with small, incidentally discovered tumors that may be benefited with a nephron-sparing approach.

Most of the available literature seems to stress the size of the tumor as the important predictor of cancer-related outcome. A recent study has disclosed excellent functional results, no local recurrences, and a 100% 5-year cancer-specific survival in patients with unilateral stage I tumors less than 4 cm in size.[8] Likewise Hafez et al reviewed the Cleveland Clinic series of 485 partial nephrectomies and reported a significant decrease in 5-year and 10-year cancer-specific survival for lesions larger than 4 cm when compared with lesions smaller than 4 cm.[9] The group also noted a statistically significant correlation between recurrence and size greater than 4 cm. Based on these data, it was proposed that stage T1 tumors (<7 cm) should be categorized as T1a, and lesions smaller than 4 cm and larger than 4 cm as T1b. Fergany et al, in an updated review of the Cleveland Clinic experience, noted a cancer-specific survival rate of 100% for unilateral tumors smaller than 4 cm.[10] The validity of tumor size as the most significant predictor of cancer-related outcome was substantiated by Lerner et al, who reported that only 3% of patients with tumors smaller than 3 cm died of renal cancer within 5 years following partial nephrectomy, compared with 20% of patients with tumors larger than 6 cm.[11] Significantly, a multivariate analysis disclosed a pronounced cancer-specific and disease-free survival advantage for patients undergoing radical nephrectomy versus partial nephrectomy for tumors larger than 4 cm.

Studies on the natural history of small renal tumors managed expectantly have demonstrated a relatively small increase in diameter, ranging from a mean 0.22 to 0.54 cm per year.[12–14] This has prompted a surveillance policy in individuals at a higher surgical risk.[15] This strategy has, however, been rendered hazardous by a recent retrospective study involving 50 tumors 3 cm or less disclosing that 38% of incidentally discovered renal cell carcinomas smaller than 3 cm in diameter had extracapsular extension (p T3) and 28% were Fuhrman grade 3/4.[16] In a more recent and detailed retrospective study involving 287 tumor-bearing kidneys, Remzi et al asserted that the aggressive potential of small renal cell carcinoma increases dramatically beyond a tumor diameter of 3 cm and they maintained that the threshold for selecting patients for a surveillance strategy should be set well under this parameter.[17]

Interestingly, the literature survey discloses few papers countering the 4 cm cut-off limit for nephron-sparing surgery in localized renal cell carcinoma with a normal contralateral kidney and extends it further to between 4 and 7 cm. Belldegrun et al compared 146 patients who underwent partial nephrectomy with a matched cohort of 125 patients who underwent radical nephrectomy after stratification of patients by tumor size and elective versus absolute indication. They documented a disease-free survival for individuals undergoing partial nephrectomy for tumors 4 to 7 cm in size equivalent to that in a matched cohort undergoing radical nephrectomy.[18] Thrasher et al likewise noted no increased incidence of recurrence for lesions of 4 to 7 cm when compared with lesions smaller than 4 cm.[19] In computing survival to tumor size, Filipas and colleagues also found no significant difference in patients with a tumor size larger or smaller than 4 cm.[20]

An increase in incidental diagnosis at an earlier age has provoked increased concerns about the long-term risk of renal insufficiency or metachronous tumor recurrence in patients undergoing radical nephrectomy. This along with the current refined surgical skill and more precise staging of renal cell carcinoma may conspire to expand the indications for elective partial nephrectomy to larger tumors in judiciously selected groups.

But currently are there any prognostic indices and nomograms to help to select those cases of large tumors who are likely to benefit by elective partial nephrectomy and as well predict long-term disease-free survival immediately after resection of clinically localized renal cell carcinoma? Currently, five prognostic nomograms are available for non-metastatic renal cell carcinoma.[21,22] A postoperative nomogram proposed by Kattan and colleagues, based on the analysis of a Memorial Sloan–Kettering database, is the most widely used model to predict treatment failure and tumor recurrence after surgery for kidney cancer.[21,22] This nomogram is designed to calculate the probability that a patient would be free from recurrences at 5 years of follow up. Predictor variables are patient symptoms, histology, tumor size, and TNM 1997 pathologic stage. In a multicentric European study it was found to be more accurate than three other models (the University of California–Los Angeles Integrated Staging System [UISS], Mayo Clinic Stage, Size, Grade, and Necrosis [SSIGN] Score, and the Yaycioglu model).[23] However, in a subsequent study the Kattan nomogram fared poorly in predicting overall renal cell carcinoma recurrence.[24]

The search for credible prognostic factors in renal cell carcinoma is still ongoing, but unfortunately no totally reliable prognostic marker has yet been established. Few developing investigational modalities such as microarray technology hold out considerable promise. Gene and/or protein expression profiles derived through microarray technology have the potential for diagnosis of a particular cancer and/or of cancer subsets, without examining the histology.[25,26] It may even be possible to predict which patients will benefit from extirpative surgical procedures.

MODES OF EXCISION

Currently a variety of surgical techniques are available for performing in-situ nephron-sparing surgery in patients with renal cell carcinoma. These include simple enucleation, segmental polar nephrectomy, wedge resection, and major transverse resection. Among the variety of surgical techniques, all except enucleation have no attendant controversies since they ensure adequate surgical margin, as demonstrated in Figures 11.1 and 11.2.

The principle of simple enucleation was first enunciated by Vermooten and it involves circumferentially incising the parenchyma around the tumor and achieving

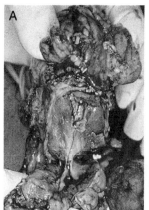
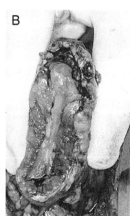

Figure 11.2 Operative photographs demonstrating lower polar nephrectomy in a left kidney.
(A) Detachment of the tumor-containing lower pole;
(B) tumor-free parenchymal defect before closure.

a plane of avascular cleavage between the pseudocapsule and the adjacent uninvolved parenchyma[27] (Figure 11.3).

The tumor is subsequently shelved out of the tumor bed with the blunt end of the scapel.[28] The presence of a distinct and uninvolved pseudocapsule is an important prerequisite for successful enucleation. This conditionality, however, cannot always be insured since some histopathologic studies have categorically demonstrated microscopic tumor infringement of the capsule in many cases.[29–31] In the current setting the technique of enucleation is best suited for patients with von Hippel–Lindau disease, which is characterized by bilateral low-stage encapsulated tumors[32] (Figure 11.4). It must, however, be noted that some series in recent literature have disclosed identical rates of cancer control between enucleation and partial nephrectomy provided the radicality of the excision is ensured through intraoperative frozen sections of the postenucleation tumor bed.[11]

SURGICAL MARGIN

It has been established that a positive surgical margin can adversely impact disease-specific survival.[19] The standard technique of partial nephrectomy, therefore, has mandated the inclusion of a 1 to 2 cm rim of normal parenchyma.[27] This strident conditionality has, however, been dented by several recent studies. In one of the studies, involving 44 patients with a mean tumor size of 3.2 cm and a mean surgical margin of 2.5 mm, 93% achieved negative margins and did not have a local recurrence with

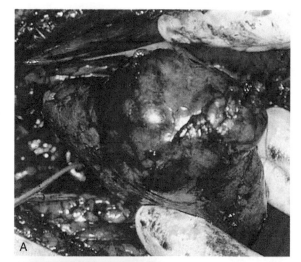
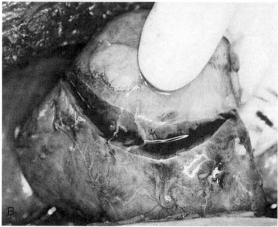

Figure 11.1 Operative photographs demonstrating
(A) a tumor on the convex border of the right kidney,
(B) wedge resection – note the inclusion of the rim of normal renal parenchyma in the excision.

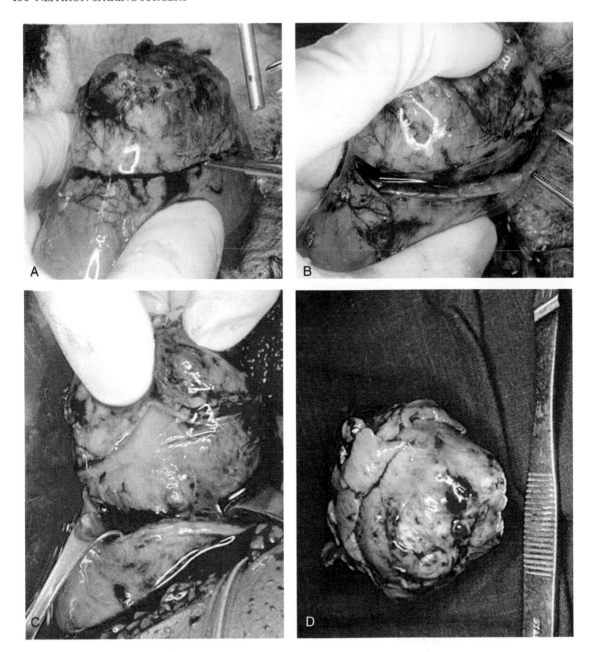

Figure 11.3 Operative photographs demonstrating the steps of encleation. (A) Initial circumferential parenchymal incision. (B) and (C) Development of cleavage between the pseudocapsule of the tumor and adjacent uninvolved parenchyma. (D) Excised tumor – the encircling rim of tissue is composed only of capsular tags.

a mean follow-up of 49 months.[33] Likewise in the Mayo Clinic series of 130 patients, the 5-year local recurrence-free survival was 97% when the tumor excision was carried out with a minimum of a 3 mm rim of normal renal tissue around the tumor.[34] Castilla et al, in their retrospective evaluation of 69 patients who underwent partial nephrectomy with a mean surgical margin of 3–5 mm, did not notice any correlation between the width of the margin and the disease progression.[35] The above studies indicate that the insistence of a minimum 1 to 2 cm margin is not mandatory provided a negative margin is insured by a frozen-section scrutiny of the

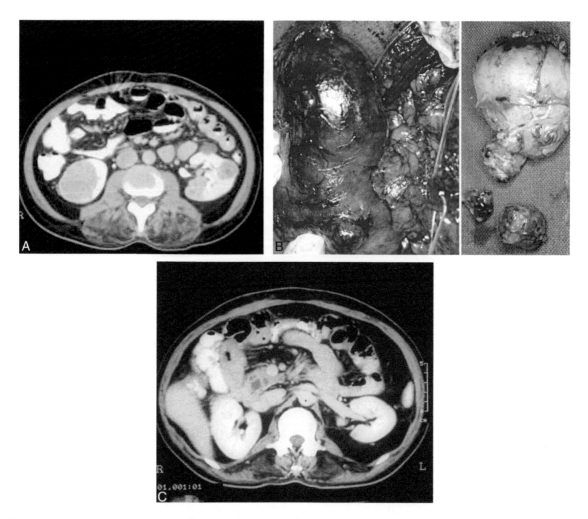

Figure 11.4 (A) Pre-operative CT of a case of von Hippel-Lindau disease showing bilateral renal tumors. (B) Intra-operative photograph of left kidney containing multiple tumors, and specimens of tumors harvested from left kidney through enucleation. (C) Post-operative CT demonstrating total bilateral clearance of tumors.

tumor bed. The current practice at our center is to provide the harvested specimen a rim of a minimum of 0.5 cm of normal renal parenchyma and this has guaranteed 100% negative surgical margins in all our cases (Figure 11.5).

TUMOR DISPOSITION

Renal tumors amenable to nephron-sparing extirpation are grouped into peripheral and central tumors. Peripheral tumors are defined as those without extension into the renal sinus and central tumors as those extending centrally into the kidney beyond the renal

medulla into the renal sinus. It was assumed that the central lesion has a propensity for metastasis in cases of incomplete excision and thus adversely impacts the cancer control. Early literature lent credence to such a contention.[27] However, subsequent studies have not substantiated this viewpoint. Hafez et al retrospectively evaluated tumor location as an independent factor and found no differences in cancer-specific survival or recurrence between central and peripheral tumors.[36] Excision of the centrally disposed lesions, though more demanding, is not beyond the realm of nephron-sparing efforts.[37] We have found regional vascular control and hypothermia extremely useful in the performance of this exacting surgery (Figure 11.6).

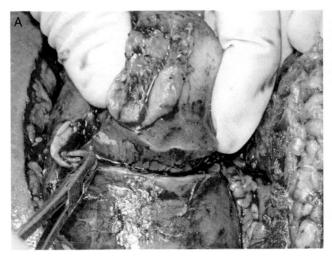

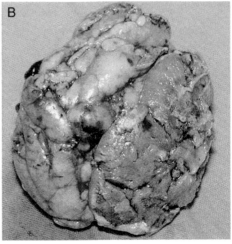

Figure 11.5 Operative photographs of a tumor excision. (A) Encircling incision to include a 0.5 cm rim of normal renal parenchyma around the tumor. (B) Specimen of the excised tumor – note the undisturbed perinephric fat on the surface and normal parenchyma covering the inferior aspect of the specimen.

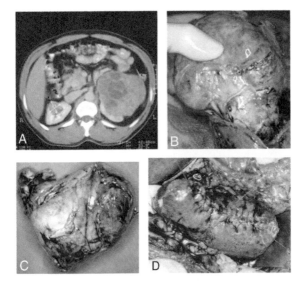

Figure 11.6 (A) CT scan demonstrating bilateral central renal tumors; the larger central lesion is seen in the left kidney. (B) Operative photograph demonstrating deep intrarenal dissection prior to excision of the tumor in the left kidney. (C) Specimen of the excised tumor – note a few satellite nodules at the base of the tumor which were also harvested along with the main tumor. (D) Postexcision closure of renal parenchyma.

Increased renal flaccidity and a bloodless surgical field produced by ischemic and hypothermic conditions aid precise intrarenal dissection and extraction of the lesion. A few central lesions may entail calyceal infringement to effect radicality of the excision and subsequent calyceal reconstruction (Figure 11.7).

Renal cell carcinoma situated at a high level and proximate to the principal renal vessels is also amenable to radical in-situ excision (Figure 11.8).

MULTICENTRICITY

It is generally conceded that multicentricity potentially increases the chances of surgical failure after partial nephrectomy. The incidence of small nodules found in kidneys removed at radical nephrectomy for renal cell carcinoma or at autopsy ranges from 4 to 25%.[5,6,38–44] Earlier literature tended to label renal tumors smaller than 3 cm as benign adenomas with meager malignant potential.[45] However, currently such small tumors are considered low-grade renal cell carcinomas.[38,46]

Increased tumor size, stage p T2 or greater, vascular invasion, and papillary or mixed histology are factors usually seen coexisting with multifocality.[38–41] Wang et al prospectively studied surgical specimens in 44 patients who underwent radical nephrectomy.[43] Their study disclosed 25% of the renal carcinomas were pathologically multifocal, 91% in primary tumors less than 5 cm. Tumor multifocality was independent of the size of the primary renal tumor but occurred with a slightly higher frequency in tumors of stage T3a or larger, even when the primary tumor was small.

There is some speculation that the satellite nodules are the result of intrarenal metastasis rather than tumor multiplicity, as the nodules have a positive relation with the size and T stage of the primary tumor.[7]

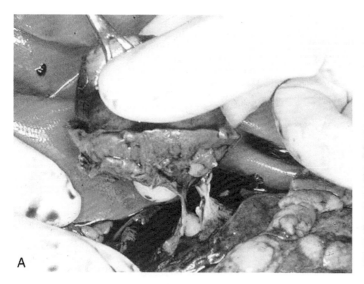
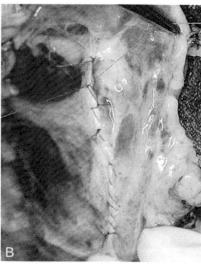

Figure 11.7 Operative photograph demonstrating (A) the excision of a central lesion along with portions of implicated calyceal groups; (B) major calyceal reconstruction after the excision of a large central lesion.

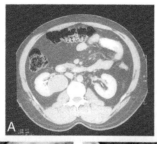
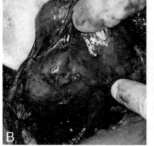
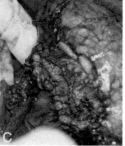

Figure 11.8 (A) CT scan showing a hilar renal cell carcinoma in the right kidney. (B) Operative photograph showing the hilar situation of the tumor. (C) Postexcision tumor base.

One disconcerting and bothersome feature of satellite nodules is that they defy preoperative CT and ultrasound evaluation and in one report the preoperative recognition of multifocality was only 22.9%.[47] Deployment of intraoperative sonography disclosed 78% of multifocal tumors and was no more accurate than the combination of preoperative CT scan and intraoperative inspection.[48]

The emergence of newer generation CT scanners, perhaps, may help in the preoperative recognition of satellite nodules more easily. The most recently produced scanners have 32 rows of detectors generating more helices and acquiring images at different slice thickness. Scanners with even more rows of detectors and image plate detectors are on the anvil and may further improve the imaging of very small structures, such as small renal masses and small renal blood vessels. Such technology may also result in less volume averaging and pixilation, factors that often limit the imaging of small renal masses.[49]

ROLE IN ADVANCED DISEASE

The imperative, relative, and elective indications for nephron-sparing surgery are clearly defined; they have a curative intent and aim for a protracted cancer-free survival. However, its role in advanced and metastatic disease is currently evolving and under scrutiny. In recent years there has been a surfeit of studies advocating the procedure in selected cases of advanced and metastatic disease and in those with vena caval involvement.[50,51] Evidently, the preservation of renal mass and adequate renal function may be critical in individuals receiving systemic cancer therapy. This is particularly so in the setting of tumor-harboring solitary kidneys with metastatic load and in those who have previously undergone contralateral radical nephrectomy for malignant disease.

REFERENCES

1. Robson CJ. Radical nephrectomy for renal cell carcinoma. J Urol 1963; 89: 37.
2. Robson CJ, Churchill BM, Anderson W. The results of radical nephrectomy for renal cell carcinoma. J Urol 1969; 101: 297.
3. Butler BP, Novick AC, Miller DP et al. Management of small unilateral renal cell carcinomas: radical vs nephron sparing surgery. Urology 1995; 45: 34.
4. Licht MR, Novick AC. Nephron sparing surgery for renal cell carcinoma. J Urol 1993; 145: 1.
5. Mukamel E, Komichezky M, Englestein D et al. Incidental small renal tumors accompanying clinically overt renal cell carcinoma. J Urol 1988; 140: 22.
6. Cheng WS, Farrow GM, Zinke H. Incidence of multicentricity in renal cell carcinoma. J Urol 1991; 146: 1221.
7. Lee SE, Kim HH. Validity of kidney preserving surgery for localized renal cell carcinoma. Eur Urol 1994; 25: 204–8.
8. Licht MR, Novick AC, Gormastic M. Nephron sparing surgery in incidental versus suspected renal cell carcinoma. J Urol 1993; 149: 1.
9. Hafez KS, Fergany AF, Novick AC. Nephron sparing surgery for localized renal cell carcinoma: impact of tumour size on patient survival, tumour recurrence and TNM staging. J Urol 1999; 162: 1930.
10. Fergany AF, Hafez KS, Novick AC. Long term results of nephron sparing surgery for localized renal cell carcinoma: 10 year follow up. J Urol 2000; 163: 442.
11. Lerner SE, Hawkins CA, Blute ML et al. Disease outcome in patients with low stage renal cell carcinoma treated with nephron sparing or radical surgery. J Urol 1996; 155: 1868.
12. Rendon RA, Stanietzky N, Panzarella T et al. The natural history of small renal masses. J Urol 2000; 164: 1143.
13. Oda T, Takahashi A, Miyao N et al. Cell proliferation, apoptosis angiogenesis and growth rate of incidently found renal cell carcinoma. Int J Urol 2003; 10: 13.
14. Kasouf W, Aprikian AG, Laplante M et al. Natural history of renal masses followed expectantly. J Urol 2004; 171: 111.
15. Renshaw A. The natural history of incidently detected small renal masses. Cancer 2004; 101: 650.
16. Hsu RM, Chan DY, Sigelman SS. Small renal cell carcinomas: correlation of size with tumour stage, nuclear grade and histologic subtype. AJR Am J Roentgenol 2004; 182: 551.
17. Remzi M, Ozsoy M, Klingler HC et al. Are small tumours harmless? Analysis of histopathological features according to tumours 4 cm or less in diameter. J Urol 2006; 176: 896–9.
18. Belldegrun A, Tsui KH, deKernion JB et al. Efficacy of nephron-sparing surgery for renal cell carcinoma: analysis based on the new 1997 tumor–node–metastasis staging system. J Clin Oncol 1999; 17: 2868.
19. Thrasher JB, Robertson JE, Paulson DF. Expanding indications for conservative renal surgery in renal cell carcinoma. Urology 1994; 43: 160.
20. Filipas D, Fichtner J, Spix C et al. Nephron sparing surgery of renal cell carcinoma with a normal opposite kidney: long term outcome in 180 patients. Urology 2000; 56: 387–92.
21. Hixson ED, Kattan MW. Nomograms are more meaningful than severity-adjusted institutional comparisons for reporting outcomes. Eur Urol 2006; 49(4): 600–3.
22. Kattan MW, Reuter V, Motzer RJ et al. A postoperative prognostic nomogram for renal cell carcinoma. J Urol 2001; 166(1): 63–7.
23. Cindolo L, Patard JJ, Chiodini P et al. Comparison of predictive accuracy of four prognostic models for nonmetastatic renal cell carcinoma after nephrectomy: a multicentre European Study. Cancer 2005; 104(7): 1362–7.
24. Hupertan V, Roupret M, Poisson JF et al. Low predictive accuracy of the Kattan postoperative nomogram for renal cell carcinoma recurrence in a population of French patients. Cancer 2006; 107(11): 2604–8.
25. Kim HL, Seligson D, Liu X et al. Molecular prognostic modelling using protein expression profile in clear cell renal cell carcinoma. J Urol 2004; 17: 436.
26. Tekahashi M, Rhodes DR, Furge KR et al. Gene expression profiling of clear cell renal cell carcinoma gene identification and prognostic classification. Proc Natl Acad Sci USA 2001; 98(17): 9754–9.
27. Vermooten V. Indications for conservative surgery in certain renal tumours: a study based on the growth pattern of clear cell carcinoma. J Urol 1950; 64: 200.
28. Graham SD Jr, Glean JF. Enucleation surgery for renal malignancy. J Urol 1979; 122: 546.
29. Marshall FF, Taxy JB, Fishman EK, Chang R. The feasibility of surgical enucleation for renal cell carcinoma. J Urol 1986; 135: 231.
30. Rosenthal CL, Kraft R, Zingg EJ. Organ-preserving surgery in renal cell carcinoma: tumour enucleation versus partial kidney resection. Eur Urol 1984; 10: 222.
31. Blackley SK, Ladaga L, Woolfitt RA et al. Ex situ study of the effectiveness of enucleation in patients with renal cell carcinoma. J Urol 1988; 140: 6.
32. Spencer WF, Novick AC, Montie JE et al. Surgical treatment of localized renal carcinoma in Von Hippel–Lindau's disease. J Urol 1988; 139: 507.
33. Sutherland SE, Resnick MI, Maclennan GT et al. Does the size of the surgical margin in partial nephrectomy for renal cell cancer really matter? J Urol 2002; 167: 61.
34. Lau WK, Blute MC, Weaver AL et al. Matched comparison of radical nephrectomy vs nephron sparing surgery in patients with unilateral renal cell carcinoma and a normal contralateral kidney. Mayo Clinic Proc 2000; 75: 1236.
35. Castilla EA, Liou LS, Abrahams NA et al. Prognostic importance of resection margin width after nephron sparing surgery for renal cell carcinoma. Urology 2002; 60: 993.
36. Hafez KS, Novick AC, Butler BP. Management of small solitary unilateral renal cell carcinomas: impact of central versus peripheral tumour location. J Urol 1998; 159: 1156.
37. Chan DY, Marshall FF. Partial nephrectomy for centrally located tumours. Urology 1999; 54: 1088.
38. Nissenkorn I, Bernheim J. Multicentricity in renal cell carcinoma. J Urol 1955; 153: 620.
39. Gohji K, Hara I, Gotoh A et al. Multifocal renal cell carcinoma in Japanese patients with tumours with maximal diameters of 50 mm or less. J Urol 1998; 159: 1144.
40. Kinouchi T, Mano M, Saiki S et al. Incidence rate of satellite tumours in renal cell carcinoma. Cancer 1999; 86: 2331.
41. Kletscher BA, Qian J, Bostwick DG et al. Prospective analysis of multifocality in renal cell carcinoma: influence of histological pattern, grade, number, size, volume and deoxyribonucleic acid ploidy. J Urol 1995; 153: 904.
42. Schilchter A, Wunderlich H, Junker K et al. Where are the limits of elective nephron sparing surgery in renal cell carcinoma? Eur Urol 2000; 37: 517.
43. Wang M, O'Toole K, Bixon R et al. The incidence of multifocal renal cell carcinoma in patients who are candidates for partial nephrectomy. J Urol 1995; 154: 968.

44. Xipell JM. The incidence of benign renal nodules (a clinico pathologic study). J Urol 1971; 106: 503.

45. Bell E. A classification of renal tumours with observations of the frequency of the various types. J Urol 1938; 39: 238.

46. Murphy GP, Mustofi FK. Histologic assessment and clinical prognosis of renal adenoma. J Urol 1970; 103: 31.

47. Schlichter A, Schubert R, Werner W et al. How accurate is diagnostic imaging in determination of size and multifocality of renal cell carcinoma as a prerequisite for nephron sparing surgery? Urol Int 2000; 64: 192.

48. Campbell SC, Fichtner J, Novick AC et al. Intraoperative evaluation of renal cell carcinoma: a prospective study of the role of ultrasonography and histopathological frozen sections. J Urol 1996; 155: 1191.

49. Lockhart ME, Smith K. Technical considerations in renal CT. In: Kenny PJ, ed. Radiologic Clinics of North America – Advances in renal imaging. Philadelphia, PA: WB Sauders Company 2003, 41(5): 863–75.

50. Angermier KW, Novick AC, Streem SB et al. Nephron-sparing surgery for renal cell carcinoma with venous involvement. J Urol 1990; 144: 1352.

51. Krishnamurthy V, Novick AC, Bukowski R. Nephron sparing surgery in patients with metastatic renal cell carcinoma. J Urol 1996; 156: 36.

12

Renal cell carcinoma: long-term outcome following nephron-sparing surgery

Murugesan Manoharan and Rajinikanth Ayyathurai

INTRODUCTION

Historically, radical nephrectomy has been considered the preferred curative treatment for localized renal cell carcinoma (RCC).[1] The nephron-sparing surgery was originally reserved for patients with solitary kidney, bilateral tumor, and renal insufficiency. With the development of modern imaging techniques renal tumors are more frequently diagnosed in asymptomatic patients. These asymptomatic locally confined lesions are often lower grade and stage. Hence the need for radical nephrectomy in such cases was challenged. This concept led to a progressive increase in the use of the nephron-sparing surgical technique, even in patients with a normal contralateral kidney.

The evolution of renal cancer surgery in the last decade has shown remarkable advancement in parenchymal sparing and minimally invasive techniques. This evolution is largely due to advances in renal imaging, improved surgical technique, better postoperative management, and availability of long-term survival data. Recent studies have established that nephron-sparing surgery provides an equally effective curative treatment with the significant advantage of a lower incidence of long-term renal insufficiency in these patients when compared with traditional radical nephrectomy.[2]

The effort to decrease operative time and patient recuperation has led to the incorporation of minimally invasive techniques in nephron-sparing surgery. Various nephron-sparing minimally invasive treatment options are being evaluated, including laparoscopic partial nephrectomy and energy ablative procedures such as radiofrequency and cryoablation. However, the technical difficulties of these procedures have limited their performance to a few centers. In this chapter, we review the long-term outcome and factors affecting the outcome of nephron-sparing surgery.

OUTCOME FACTORS

Surgical expertise and technologic advancement have established nephron-sparing surgery as a safe and effective surgical procedure. Nephron-sparing surgery aims at complete cancer eradication while preserving as much normal renal parenchyma as possible. Various clinical, pathologic, and operative factors are recognized to affect the outcome of nephron-sparing procedures. Table 12.1 illustrates the important factors influencing the outcome of nephron-sparing surgery.

SOLITARY AND NORMAL CONTRALATERAL KIDNEY

The absolute indications of nephron-sparing surgery are tumor arising from a solitary kidney, bilateral tumors, and significant renal insufficiency. Many early series reported the outcome of nephron-sparing surgery in patients who would otherwise become anephric after radical nephrectomy. Maximal preservation of unaffected renal parenchyma with a view to minimize long-term morbidity has led to the concept of elective nephron-sparing surgery in patients with a normal contralateral kidney. Uzzo and Novick reviewed 1833 nephron-sparing surgery reported in the literature since 1980 and showed the mean 5-year cancer-specific survival to range between 72 and 100%.[3] Table 12.2 shows the 5-year outcome of nephron-sparing surgery in published series. Fergany et al reported the outcome of 107 nephron-sparing surgery patients with a minimum follow-up of 10 years. Of these patients, 90% underwent nephron-sparing surgery for an absolute indication such as solitary kidney. Cancer-specific survival in this group was 88% and 73% at 5 and 10 years, respectively.[4] The Mayo Clinic reported 81% and 64% cancer-specific

Table 12.1 Factors affecting the outcome of nephron-sparing surgery for renal cell carcinoma

Solitary kidney
Tumor size > 4 cm (>7 cm?)
Positive margin status
Multiple tumors
Tumor stage > T2
Nuclear grade 3
Clear cell histology

survival at 5 and 10 years for 76 patients who underwent nephron-sparing surgery for RCC in solitary kidney.[5] On the other hand, Herr reviewed the Memorial Sloan–Kettering Cancer Center (MSKCC) series of nephron-sparing surgery for renal carcinoma with normal contralateral kidney. They reported a 97.5% disease-free survival with a minimum of 10 years' mean follow-up.[6] Delakas et al reported on 118 cases of elective nephron-sparing surgery from a European multicenter review with 10- and 15-year cancer specific outcome of 96.4%.[7] Table 12.3 shows the reported outcome from various elective nephron-sparing surgery series. The overall cancer-specific survival rates are higher in series with elective nephron-sparing surgery when compared with the absolutely indicated series.

TUMOR SIZE

The staging system of the RCC has gone through several modifications over the last few decades. The 1987 AJCC classification defined stage T1 as tumor size ≤ 2.5 cm.[8] The 1997 AJCC revised stage T1 as tumor size ≤ 7 cm.[9,10] Subsequently in 2003, T1 was further subdivided into T1a ≤ 4 cm and T1b ≥ 4 but ≤ 7 cm. Review of long-term data on nephron-sparing surgery shows size of the tumor is the most important predictor of cancer-related outcome.[2,4,11,12]

The current evidence support elective nephron-sparing surgery for renal masses of 4 cm or smaller in their greatest dimension. Hafez et al studied the impact of tumor size on patient survival and tumor recurrence following nephron-sparing surgery for localized RCC. They reviewed 485 nephron-sparing surgeries and reported that the 5- and 10-year cancer-specific survival in patients with tumors ≤4 cm was 96%, and 90%, respectively, and in patients with tumors of size > 4 cm it was 86% and 66%, respectively. They concluded

cancer-free survival is significantly better in patients with tumors of 4 cm or less compared with large tumors. They also showed a significant correlation between recurrence and tumor size greater than 4 cm.[11] Fergany et al reviewed 107 patients with nephron-sparing surgery and concluded that patients with tumors greater than 4 cm were significantly more likely to die of disease than those with tumors less than 4 cm. They further reported that, from the Cox proportional hazard model, for each 1 cm increase in tumor size the risk of death increased by 20%.[4] Data from the Mayo Clinic and MSKCC reported 91% and 95% 5-year disease-free survival, respectively, for patients undergoing nephron-sparing surgery for RCC ≤ 4 cm.[12,13] Becker et al reviewed 216 patients and suggested nephron-sparing surgery should be the gold standard for tumors less than 4 cm in size.[14] Though the 4 cm cut off for T1a is well accepted, many clinicians proposed nephron-sparing procedure for tumors ranging from 4.5 to 5.5 cm.[15–17]

As data on nephron-sparing surgery accumulated, the possibility of expanding the indications of nephron-sparing surgery to tumors between 4 and 7 cm was explored by many investigators. Leibovich et al compared 91 nephron-sparing surgeries with 841 radical nephrectomies performed for unilateral RCC of size between 4 and 7 cm. They did not observe any statistically significant differences in cancer-specific or metastasis-free survival between patients treated with nephron-sparing surgery and radical nephrectomy. They concluded that these tumors can be treated by elective nephron-sparing surgery when they have an exophytic growth pattern and present minimal risk to the collecting system.[18] Becker et al reported 10- and 15-year cancer-specific survival probabilities of 100% for 69 patients who underwent nephron-sparing surgery for tumors larger than 4 cm. They emphasized the importance of patient selection on the basis of tumor localization and technical feasibility in order to achieve long-term cancer control.[19] Similar findings were published by Belldegrun et al suggesting elective nephron-sparing surgery for tumors less than 7 cm.[20] However, further long-term results are awaited before these recommendations are incorporated into routine practice.

TUMOR LOCATION

Early reports have examined tumor location and its association with cancer-related outcome in patients with RCC and suggested centrally located tumors had a greater risk for metastasis at presentation. Hafez et al studied 86 patients who underwent nephron-sparing surgery for tumor size less than 4 cm and reported 5-year disease-free survival rates of 97% and 100% for peripheral and

Table 12.2 Outcome analysis in patients undergoing nephron-sparing surgery for renal cell carcinoma

Studies	No. of patients	Mean follow-up	Cancer-specific survival (%)	Local recurrence (%)
Marberger et al[60]	72	NA	78	8
Bazeed et al[61]	51	36	96	4
Carini et al[62]	35	46	89	3
Morgan and Zincke[63]	104	60	89	6
Moll et al[64]	142	35	98	1.4
Lee et al[10]	79	40	96	0
Steinbach et al[65]	121	47	90	4.1
Lerner et al[9]	185	44	89	5.9
Hafez et al[8]	485	47	92	3.2
Belldegrun et al[17]	146	74	93	2.7
Barbalias et al[66]	41	59	98	7.3
Fergany et al[4]	107	120	88	4
Pahernik et al[30]	381	80	98.5	2.3
Leibovich et al[15]	91	107	98	5.4
Becker et al[16]	368	74	100	5.8
Zigeuner et al[67]	114	80	94	6.1

Table 12.3 Outcome analysis of elective nephron-sparing surgery series

Study	No. of patients	Mean follow-up	Mean tumor size	Cancer specific survival (%)	Local recurrence (%)
Herr[6]	70	120	3	98	1.5
Hafez et al[8]	45	47	<4	100	0
Delakas et al[7]	118	102	3.3	97.3	3.9
Van Poppel et al[68]	51	75	3	98	0
Moll et al[64]	98	35	4	100	1
Lerner et al[9]	54	44	≤4	92	5.6
Steinbach et al[65]	72	47	3.3	94	2.7
Bazeed et al[61]	23	36	3.3	100	0

centrally located tumors, respectively. They concluded central tumors had no statistically different outcome on 5-year cancer-specific survival or tumor recurrence when compared with peripheral tumors.[21] However, nephron-sparing surgery is technically more challenging in central lesions. The authors concluded that there was no inherent variation in biologic behavior between central and peripheral lesions. The decision to perform nephron-sparing surgery in a centrally located tumor is based on the technical feasibility as the outcomes are similar.

MARGIN STATUS

Local tumor recurrence remains the main concern of nephron-sparing surgery and it may be due to incomplete

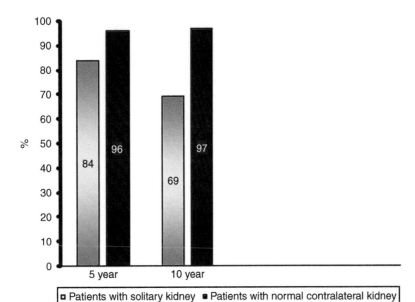

Figure 12.1 5-year and 10-year cancer-specific survival following nephron-sparing surgery.

resection of primary tumor, occult multicentric disease, or a new occurrence. It is widely accepted that tumor excision with a surrounding margin of normal parenchyma is the safe approach to ensure complete removal of malignancy during nephron-sparing surgery. Although earlier reports have suggested including a 1 cm rim of normal parenchyma in the resected specimen, generally no agreement has been reached among clinicians about the amount of normal parenchyma to be removed with the tumor. Castilla et al reviewed 69 localized RCC patients who had undergone nephron-sparing surgery and concluded that the width of the resection margin after nephron-sparing surgery for RCC does not correlate with long-term disease progression. They also emphasized that the histologic tumor-free margin of resection, irrespective of the width of the margin, is sufficient to achieve the expected cancer control.[22] Lau et al reviewed the Mayo Clinic series where each partial nephrectomy was performed with a margin of at least 3 mm of normal parenchyma around the tumor followed by a frozen section biopsy of the tumor bed. They achieved a 5-year local recurrence-free survival of 97%.[2] These data suggest that excision of all gross tumor, followed by a series of frozen section biopsies obtained randomly from the renal resection margin to confirm the absence of malignancy in the remaining portion of kidney, is the safest practice.[23] Few recent studies have reported comparable rates of cancer control with tumor enucleation.[24] However, many histopathologic reports have demonstrated microscopic tumor penetration of the pseudocapsule in the enucleated specimens. After reviewing

the literature, we conclude that complete resection with a negative margin is the critical factor in outcome rather than the amount of normal parenchyma excised.

MULTIPLE TUMORS

The risk of multifocal tumor raises a serious concern about the widespread application of the nephron-sparing technique. A high incidence of multicentric RCC has been reported in genetic syndromes such as the Von Hippel–Lindau syndrome. The incidence of multifocality in sporadic RCC is less well understood. A review of published data from radical nephrectomy and autopsy specimen shows a wide range in incidence of multifocal RCC from 6.5% to 28%.[25-27] Factors influencing the multifocality are an increase in tumor size, T stage, tumor histology, and grade. Papillary and mixed pattern RCCs are known to be associated with a higher incidence of multicentric disease than other histologic variants.[28-30] Many investigators have shown that the risk of multifocal disease increases with larger tumors, particularly stage pT2 or greater. After a cumulative review of 1000 cases Uzzo and Novick reported that the incidence of multifocality was 5% when the primary tumor was 4 cm or less.[3] With the available data the relationship of multifocality to local recurrence is not clearly understood. However, it is very low when primary tumor is less than 4 cm. A preoperative CT scan and intraoperative ultrasound have been shown to be sensitive in localizing the tumors in kidney. A recent prospective study reported that 78% of multifocal tumors were identified by intraoperative ultrasound, however it was not more sensitive than the combination of CT scan and intraoperative inspection.[31]

PATHOLOGIC VARIABLES

It is well acknowledged that the outcome of renal cancer surgery is influenced by the histologic subtype of RCC.[16] Studies have shown that the clear cell type is more aggressive than other subtypes such as papillary and chromophobe RCC. Krejci et al reviewed 344 cases of nephron-sparing surgery for RCC and concluded that patients with the clear cell subtype have a significantly poor cancer-specific survival and are more likely to die of RCC compared to those with papillary or chromophobe subtypes.[32] Pahernik et al reported 25 years of experience of elective nephron-sparing surgery among 715 patients where 88% of local recurrences belonged to clear cell variants.[33] In addition, the presence of histologic tumor necrosis was significantly associated with death from clear cell and chromophobe RCC.[34] Ghavamian et al reported no distant metastases with papillary or chromophobe RCC in their cohort of 63 patients who underwent nephron-sparing surgery for RCC in solitary kidney.[5] However, a rare variant, cystic clear cell type, has not been reported to be as aggressive as traditional clear cell RCC.[34] Corica et al reported 24 cases of this rare variant and suggested partial nephrectomy as a treatment option for the cystic clear cell subtype.[35]

TUMOR STAGE AND NUCLEAR GRADE

Ghavamian et al showed that tumor stage and nuclear grade were the significant predictors of distant metastasis and death due to RCC in patients treated with nephron-sparing surgery. Their multivariate model also concluded that patients with pT3b or pT4 were 5 times more likely to develop metastases or die from RCC than those with stage pT1 or pT2 tumor. Patients with tumor nuclear grade 3 were 3 times more likely to have distant metastases or disease-specific death than those with grade 1 or 2 tumors.[5] Castilla et al found a similar predictive value with Fuhrman nuclear grade and tumor stage in patients who underwent nephron-sparing surgery.[22] Fergany et al reported that patients with stage T3a and T3b tumors were 4 and 8 times, respectively, more likely to die of disease than those with stage T1 tumors.[4] Cheville et al reported tumor stage, nuclear grade, and sarcomatoid component were significantly associated with death due to RCC.[34] Due to logistic

reasons there are no studies comparing the nephron-sparing procedures with radical nephrectomy for tumor stage ≥ T3. The decision to perform a nephron-sparing procedure in these settings relies on patient assessment and the surgeon's discretion.

SPECIAL SITUATIONS – HEREDITARY RENAL TUMORS

Genetic conditions such as the Von Hippel–Lindau (VHL) syndrome, hereditary papillary RCC, and the Birt–Hogg–Dubet syndrome are well known to predispose patients to recurrent renal neoplasms at a younger age. The treatment strategy for patients with hereditary RCC differs significantly from sporadic RCC because of their tendency to be bilateral, multifocal, and often recurrent. The benefit of nephron-sparing surgery in these patients is preserving renal function and avoiding dialysis. These patients have a high risk of local recurrences and may need multiple nephron-sparing surgical procedures. In a multicenter study, 49 patients with VHL syndrome who were treated with nephron-sparing surgery were reported to have 100% and 81% survival at 5 and 10 years, respectively.[36] With 68 months of mean follow-up, this study reported 85% local recurrence at 10 years. These data call attention to the potential of these tumors to recur and the importance of meticulous surveillance after nephron-sparing surgery in these patients.[36–38] Similarly, Walther et al evaluated 52 patients with VHL syndrome and RCC and recommended observation for tumors less than 3 cm.[39] Current data suggest that nephron-sparing surgery is feasible in most patients with VHL disease, which may preserve renal function without compromising on cancer control. However, lifelong diligent surveillance is mandatory.

ALLOGRAFT KIDNEY

De novo RCC is a recognized complication of renal transplantation with a reported incidence of 4.6%.[40] Transplant nephrectomy for allograft RCC renders the patient anephric with an immediate need for dialysis. Recent reports have suggested that nephron-sparing surgery is an optimal choice for RCC of allograft kidney whenever feasible. Ribal et al reviewed 14 cases of allograft RCC with a mean follow-up of 32 months and reported no local recurrence, renal failure, or distant dissemination. Although technically challenging, current data suggest that nephron-sparing surgery may provide acceptable cancer control for tumors less than 4 cm in diameter without impaired graft function.[41]

MINIMALLY INVASIVE APPROACH

Open nephron-sparing surgery has become an accepted treatment for carefully selected RCC. Although nephron-sparing surgery preserves the normal renal parenchyma, it is not associated with a decrease in hospital stay or duration of surgery when compared with radical nephrectomy. This has led to the development of laparoscopic partial nephrectomy for treatment of RCC. Though few centers excel in this procedure, the reported cumulative experience comprises less than 500 cases with variable results. This procedure, either in the transperitoneal or the retroperitoneal approach, poses several challenges, including adequate margin of resection, hemostasis, preventing urine leakage, and tumor spillage. Despite numerous technologic additions such as the argon beam coagulator, harmonic scalpel, fibrin glue, and gelatin sponges major complications have occurred necessitating nephrectomy.[42] Recently a large series from the Cleveland Clinic showed that laparoscopic partial nephrectomy is a technically feasible procedure for selected patients with renal tumor. They reported operative results from 275 laparoscopic partial nephrectomies with a mean follow-up of 11 months. This study reported a mean surgery duration of 180 minutes, mean blood loss of 125 ml, and an average hospital stay of 2 days. They also described the laparoscopic partial nephrectomy as a challenging operation with potential for serious complications.[43] With increasing surgical experience and standardization of the surgical steps the immediate outcome of laparoscopic nephron-sparing surgery may improve, until then it must be undertaken by a team with considerable experience in advanced urologic laparoscopy. Long-term oncologic outcomes are not yet available for minimally invasive nephron-sparing procedures.

OTHER ENERGY SOURCES

In a separate yet related development of nephron-sparing surgery is the application of various energy sources to achieve oncologic control in selected renal tumors. Among the various ablative techniques, cryoablation remains the best reported. Cryoablation has been used in open laparoscopic as well as percutaneous approaches. The Cleveland Clinic series reported results from 50 patients with single, small (<4 cm), solid, peripheral renal tumors without involvement of the renal collecting system who underwent laparoscopic cyroablation.[44] There was no case with local recurrence with follow-up of up to 3 years. Rukstalis et al reported 29 patients who had open cryoablation with 91% complete response on a mean follow-up of 16 months.[45] However there

were more complications such as renal failure and conversion to nephrectomy with open cryoablation. Shingleton et al reported no local recurrence after percutanoeus cryoablation in 20 patients with a mean follow-up of 9 months.[46] A major concern of cryoablation is the lack of histologic documentation of complete destruction of tumor. Until longer follow-up is available these ablative techniques are reserved for special situations such as small exophytic tumors in patients who are poor surgical candidates.

Newer energy resources for tumor ablation include radiofrequency ablation (RFA), high-intensity focused ultrasound (HIFU), LASER interstitial thermotherapy (LITT), microwave thermotherapy (MT), and photon irradiation. The projected benefits of these minimally invasive therapies include parenchymal preservation and shorter recovery leading to reduced hospital stay. These modalities may be suitable either for minimally invasive or complete extracorporeal tumor ablation. RFA is the second most popular to cyroablation, with a relatively good number of cases reported. The largest series of 73 tumors in 62 patients, reported by McGovern et al, showed complete response in all tumors less than 3 cm and 81% response in tumors over 3 cm.[47,48] However, more recent reports cautioned about the presence of viable foci of tumor mostly at the margin of ablation.[49–51] The significance of these findings will be determined as longer follow-up and larger series become available. HIFU offers the potential advantage of being completely non-invasive, however only very few cases have been reported so far. Microwave thermotherapy and LITT are still in the experimental phase. More data on safety profile, ideal energy settings, histologic effect on renal tissue, clinical efficacy, and accuracy are expected before implementation of these techniques.

ADVANCED RCC

The role of nephron-sparing surgery as a symptomatic therapy in the setting of locally advanced or metastatic RCC has been reported. Nephron-sparing surgery is primarily focused to avoid or postpone renal replacement therapy in such patients. Krishnamurthi et al reported on the clinical outcome of 15 patients with metastatic RCC who underwent nephron-sparing surgery with surgical or systemic treatment for metastasis.[52] Angermeier et al reported on 9 patients with RCC involving the venous system who underwent nephron-sparing surgery.[53] Both the above mentioned studies reported technical success and preservation of renal function after nephron-sparing surgery in these circumstances. These data suggest nephron-sparing surgery may occasionally be an effective and acceptable treatment for locally advanced or completely resected metastatic RCC with preservation of renal function.

LONG-TERM RENAL FUNCTION

Many studies have evaluated the long-term effect of renal surgery on the function of the remaining kidney. Though many reports have shown an increased incidence of hypertension, protenuria, and renal insufficiency in patients with a solitary kidney, the incidence of endstage renal disease and the need for dialysis are not significantly different from that of the general population.[3] Adaptive hyperfiltration by the glomerular apparatus has been shown when there is a greater than 50% loss of renal tissue.[54] Novick et al reported an association between residual renal tissue and the development of proteinuria, which is the hallmark of hyperfiltration injury.[55] Fergany et al reported 10-year functional results of 96 patients who underwent nephron-sparing surgery for absolute indications. Postoperatively, 7 (6.5%) of the patients progressed to renal failure and required renal replacement therapy at an average of 8.2 years, of which 5 had preoperative renal dysfunction.[4] A series from the Mayo Clinic retrospectively compared long-term renal function in patients who underwent radical nephrectomy ($n = 126$) and elective nephron-sparing surgery ($n = 130$). At 10 years, the cumulative incidence of chronic renal insufficiency was 22.4% for radical nephrectomy and 11.6% for nephron-sparing

surgery.[2] These data may suggest that patients with absolute indications for nephron-sparing surgery are at higher risk for long-term renal insufficiency. In addition, elective nephron-sparing surgery may have a reduced risk of developing proteinuria and chronic renal injury when compared with radical nephrectomy.

SUMMARY

Recent data have demonstrated no significant difference in cancer-specific and metastasis-free survival between patients treated with nephron-sparing surgery and radical nephrectomy for small renal tumors.[2,12,13] However, there are very few published prospective reports comparing nephron-sparing surgery with radical nephrectomy. Table 12.4 lists the studies which retrospectively compared the two surgical procedures controling age, gender, and tumor stage. Moreover, the complication rates, morbidity, and mortality are similar in nephron-sparing surgery and radical nephrectomy.[56,57] The prospective randomized European Organization for Research and Treatment of Cancer (EORTC) intergroup phase 3 study randomized 541 patients into elective nephron-sparing surgery ($n = 286$) and radical nephrectomy ($n = 273$) for low-stage RCC. On comparing the complications they concluded that elective nephron-sparing surgery is a safe choice for small, easily resectable, incidentally discovered RCC with slightly higher complication rates than after radical nephrectomy.[58] The long-term oncologic

Table 12.4 Outcome analysis between radical nephrectomy and nephron-sparing surgery				
References	No. of patients undergoing RN/NSS	5-year cancer-specific survival (RN)	5-year cancer-specific survival (NSS)	Mean follow-up
Lee et al[10]	183/79	95	95	38
Lerner et al[9]	209/185	89	89	120
Lau et al[2]	164/164	97	98	60
Butler et al[55]	42/46	97	100	48
Belldegrun et al[17]	125/108	91	98	48
McKiernan et al[69]	173/117	99	96	26*
Barbalias et al[66]	48/41	98	97	59
Indudhara et al[56]	71/35	94	91	41*
D'Armiento et al[70]	21/19	96	96	70
Leibovich et al[15]	91/841	98	86	107

*Median.

results are eagerly awaited from this study which may confirm nephron-sparing surgery as an acceptable approach for small asymptomatic RCC. Alongside comparable cancer control, the major perceived benefit of partial nephrectomy is preservation of normal renal parenchyma. Many studies have reported a statistically significant reduced risk of chronic renal impairment in patients undergoing elective nephron-sparing surgery compared to radical nephrectomy.[2,59,60] There are a few reports where nephron-sparing surgery has been shown to result in a better quality of life, reduced hospital stay, and improved cost-effectiveness when compared with radical nephrectomy.[57,61,62] Poulakis et al reported that quality of life correlates proportionally with size of tumor and is significantly better for patients undergoing elective nephron-sparing surgery for tumors of less than 4 cm.[63]

In conclusion, nephron-sparing surgery is a safe and effective treatment choice for selected patients with localized RCC. As the data accumulate, the indications for elective nephron-sparing surgery may expand to include unifocal RCC more than 4 cm in size with a normal contralateral kidney. The reported cancer-specific survival for these patients has been 90–100% with a low recurrence rate of 0–3%. The recent long-term data show comparable cancer control rates between nephron-sparing surgery and radical nephrectomy, with a remarkable benefit of decreased risk of chronic renal insufficiency among nephron-sparing surgery patients. The future of nephron-sparing surgery will be dominated by minimally invasive procedures such as laparoscopic and robotic partial nephrectomy and various energy-based ablative techniques, that will significantly reduce the morbidity.

REFERENCES

1. Robson CJ. Radical nephrectomy for renal cell carcinoma. J Urol 1963; 89: 37–42.
2. Lau WK, Blute ML, Weaver AL et al. Matched comparison of radical nephrectomy vs nephron-sparing surgery in patients with unilateral renal cell carcinoma and a normal contralateral kidney. Mayo Clin Proc 2000; 75: 1236–42.
3. Uzzo RG, Novick AC. Nephron sparing surgery for renal tumors: indications, techniques and outcomes. J Urol 2001; 166: 6–18.
4. Fergany AF, Hafez KS, Novick AC: Long-term results of nephron sparing surgery for localized renal cell carcinoma: 10-year followup. J Urol 2000; 163: 442–5.
5. Ghavamian R, Cheville JC, Lohse CM et al. Renal cell carcinoma in the solitary kidney: an analysis of complications and outcome after nephron sparing surgery. J Urol 2002; 168: 454–9.
6. Herr HW. Partial nephrectomy for unilateral renal carcinoma and a normal contralateral kidney: 10-year followup. J Urol 1999; 161: 33–4; discussion 34–5.
7. Delakas D, Karyotis I, Daskalopoulos G et al. Nephron-sparing surgery for localized renal cell carcinoma with a normal contralateral kidney: a European three-center experience. Urology 2002; 60: 998–1002.
8. Harmer M. TNM classification of malignant tumors, 3rd edition. Geneva: International Union Against Cancer, 1978.
9. Fleming ID, Cooper JS, Henson DE et al. AJCC cancer staging manual, 5th edition. Philadelphia: Lippincott-Raven Publishers: 231–2, 1997.
10. Guinan P, Sobin LH, Algaba F et al. TNM staging of renal cell carcinoma. Cancer 1997; 80: 992–3.
11. Hafez KS, Fergany AF, Novick AC. Nephron sparing surgery for localized renal cell carcinoma: impact of tumor size on patient survival, tumor recurrence and TNM staging. J Urol 1999; 162: 1930–3.
12. Lerner SE, Hawkins CA, Blute ML et al. Disease outcome in patients with low stage renal cell carcinoma treated with nephron sparing or radical surgery. J Urol 1996; 155: 1868–73.
13. Lee CT, Katz J, Shi W et al. Surgical management of renal tumors 4 cm or less in a contemporary cohort. J Urol 2000; 163: 730–6.
14. Becker F, Siemer S, Humke U et al. Elective nephron sparing surgery should become standard treatment for small unilateral renal cell carcinoma: long-term survival data of 216 patients. Eur Urol 2006; 49: 308–13.
15. Ficarra V, Prayer-Galetti T, Novara G et al. Tumor-size breakpoint for prognostic stratification of localized renal cell carcinoma. Urology 2004; 63: 235–9; discussion 239–40.
16. Lau WK, Cheville JC, Blute ML et al. Prognostic features of pathologic stage T1 renal cell carcinoma after radical nephrectomy. Urology 2002; 59: 532–7.
17. Zisman A, Pantuck AJ, Chao D et al. Reevaluation of the 1997 TNM classification for renal cell carcinoma: T1 and T2 cutoff point at 4.5 rather than 7 cm better correlates with clinical outcome. J Urol 2001; 166: 54–8.
18. Leibovich BC, Blute ML, Cheville JC et al. Nephron sparing surgery for appropriately selected renal cell carcinoma between 4 and 7 cm results in outcome similar to radical nephrectomy. J Urol 2004; 171: 1066–70.
19. Becker F, Siemer S, Hack M et al. Excellent long-term cancer control with elective nephron-sparing surgery for selected renal cell carcinomas measuring more than 4 cm. Eur Urol 2006; 49: 1058–63; discussion 1063–4.
20. Belldegrun A, Tsui KH, deKernion JB et al. Efficacy of nephron-sparing surgery for renal cell carcinoma: analysis based on the new 1997 tumor–node–metastasis staging system. J Clin Oncol 1999; 17: 2868–75.
21. Hafez KS, Novick AC, Butler BP. Management of small solitary unilateral renal cell carcinomas: impact of central versus peripheral tumor location. J Urol 1998; 159: 1156–60.
22. Castilla EA, Liou LS, Abrahams NA. Prognostic importance of resection margin width after nephron-sparing surgery for renal cell carcinoma. Urology 2002; 60: 993–7.
23. Novick AC. Nephron-sparing surgery for renal cell carcinoma. Annu Rev Med 2002; 53: 393–407.
24. Lapini A, Serni S, Minervini A et al. Progression and long-term survival after simple enucleation for the elective treatment of renal cell carcinoma: experience in 107 patients. J Urol 2005; 174: 57–60; discussion 60.
25. Kinouchi T, Mano M, Saiki S et al. Incidence rate of satellite tumors in renal cell carcinoma. Cancer 1999; 86: 2331–6.
26. Miller J, Fischer C, Freese R et al. Nephron-sparing surgery for renal cell carcinoma – is tumor size a suitable parameter for indication? Urology 1999; 54: 988–93.
27. Oya M, Nakamura K, Baba S et al. Intrarenal satellites of renal cell carcinoma: histopathologic manifestation and clinical implication. Urology 1995; 46: 161–4.
28. Delahunt B, Eble JN. Papillary renal cell carcinoma: a clinico-pathologic and immunohistochemical study of 105 tumors. Mod Pathol 1997; 10: 537–44.

29. Ornstein DK, Lubensky IA, Venzon D et al. Prevalence of microscopic tumors in normal appearing renal parenchyma of patients with hereditary papillary renal cancer. J Urol 2000; 163: 431–3.

30. Kletscher BA, Qian J, Bostwick DG et al. Prospective analysis of multifocality in renal cell carcinoma: influence of histological pattern, grade, number, size, volume and deoxyribonucleic acid ploidy. J Urol 1995; 153: 904–6.

31. Campbell SC, Fichtner J, Novick AC et al. Intraoperative evaluation of renal cell carcinoma: a prospective study of the role of ultrasonography and histopathological frozen sections. J Urol 1996; 155: 1191–5.

32. Krejci KG, Blute ML, Cheville JC et al. Nephron-sparing surgery for renal cell carcinoma: clinicopathologic features predictive of patient outcome. Urology 2003; 62: 641–6.

33. Pahernik S, Roos F, Hampel C et al. Nephron sparing surgery for renal cell carcinoma with normal contralateral kidney: 25 years of experience. J Urol 2006; 175: 2027–31.

34. Cheville JC, Lohse CM, Zincke H et al. Comparisons of outcome and prognostic features among histologic subtypes of renal cell carcinoma. Am J Surg Pathol 2003; 27: 612–24.

35. Corica FA, Iczkowski KA, Cheng L et al. Cystic renal cell carcinoma is cured by resection: a study of 24 cases with long-term followup. J Urol 1999; 161: 408–11.

36. Steinbach F, Novick AC, Zincke H et al. Treatment of renal cell carcinoma in von Hippel–Lindau disease: a multicenter study. J Urol 1995; 153: 1812–6.

37. Novick AC, Streem SB. Long-term followup after nephron sparing surgery for renal cell carcinoma in von Hippel–Lindau disease. J Urol 1992; 147: 1488–90.

38. Shinohara N, Nonomura K, Harabayashi T et al. Nephron sparing surgery for renal cell carcinoma in von Hippel–Lindau disease. J Urol 1995; 154: 2016–19.

39. Walther MM, Choyke PL, Glenn G et al. Renal cancer in families with hereditary renal cancer: prospective analysis of a tumor size threshold for renal parenchymal sparing surgery. J Urol 1999; 161: 1475–9.

40. Penn I. Occurrence of cancers in immunosuppressed organ transplant recipients. Clin Transpl 1998; 147–58.

41. Ribal MJ, Rodriguez F, Musquera M et al. Nephron-sparing surgery for renal cancer: a choice of treatment in an allograft kidney. Transplant Proc 2006; 38: 1359–62.

42. Mabjeesh NJ, Avidor Y, Matzkin H. Emerging nephron sparing treatments for kidney tumors: a continuum of modalities from energy ablation to laparoscopic partial nephrectomy. J Urol 2004; 171: 553–60.

43. Desai MM, Gill IS. Laparoscopic partial nephrectomy for tumour: current status at the Cleveland Clinic. BJU Int 2005; 95(Suppl 2): 41–5.

44. Gill IS, Novick AC, Meraney AM et al. Laparoscopic renal cryoablation in 32 patients. Urology 2000; 56: 748–53.

45. Rukstalis DB, Khorsandi M, Garcia FU et al. Clinical experience with open renal cryoablation. Urology 2001; 57: 34–9.

46. Shingleton WB, Sewell PE Jr. Percutaneous renal tumor cryoablation with magnetic resonance imaging guidance. J Urol 2001; 165: 773–6.

47. Ankem MK, Nakada SY. Needle-ablative nephron-sparing surgery. BJU Int 2005; 95(Suppl 2): 46–51.

48. McGovern FJ. Percutaneous ablation of renal cancer: what is best? AUA annual meeting, Plenary session, Chicago, 2003.

49. Hsu TH, Fidler ME, Gill IS. Radiofrequency ablation of the kidney: acute and chronic histology in porcine model. Urology 2000; 56: 872–5.

50. Michaels MJ, Rhee HK, Mourtzinos AP et al. Incomplete renal tumor destruction using radio frequency interstitial ablation. J Urol 2002; 168: 2406–9; discussion 2409–10.

51. Rendon RA, Kachura JR, Sweet JM et al. The uncertainty of radio frequency treatment of renal cell carcinoma: findings at immediate and delayed nephrectomy. J Urol 2002; 167: 1587–92.

52. Krishnamurthi V, Novick AC, Bukowski R. Nephron sparing surgery in patients with metastatic renal cell carcinoma. J Urol 1996; 156: 36–9.

53. Angermeier KW, Novick AC, Streem SB et al. Nephron-sparing surgery for renal cell carcinoma with venous involvement. J Urol 1990; 144: 1352–5.

54. Brenner BM. Hemodynamically mediated glomerular injury and the progressive nature of kidney disease. Kidney Int 1983; 23: 647–55.

55. Novick AC, Gephardt G, Guz B et al. Long-term follow-up after partial removal of a solitary kidney. N Engl J Med 1991; 325: 1058–62.

56. Corman JM, Penson DF, Hur K et al. Comparison of complications after radical and partial nephrectomy: results from the National Veterans Administration Surgical Quality Improvement Program. BJU Int 2000; 86: 782–9.

57. Shekarriz B, Upadhyay J, Shekarriz H et al. Comparison of costs and complications of radical and partial nephrectomy for treatment of localized renal cell carcinoma. Urology 2002; 59: 211–15.

58. Van Poppel H, Da Pozzo L, Albrecht W et al. A prospective randomized EORTC Intergroup Phase 3 study comparing the complications of elective nephron-sparing surgery and radical nephrectomy for low-stage renal cell carcinoma. Eur Urol 2006: doi.10.1016/j.eururo.2006.11.0132006.

59. Butler BP, Novick AC, Miller DP et al. Management of small unilateral renal cell carcinomas: radical versus nephron-sparing surgery. Urology 1995; 45: 34–40; discussion 40–1.

60. Indudhara R, Bueschen AJ, Urban DA et al. Nephron-sparing surgery compared with radical nephrectomy for renal tumors: current indications and results. South Med J 1997; 90: 982–5.

61. Clark PE, Schover LR, Uzzo RG et al. Quality of life and psychological adaptation after surgical treatment for localized renal cell carcinoma: impact of the amount of remaining renal tissue. Urology 2001; 57: 252–6.

62. Uzzo RG, Wei JT, Hafez K et al. Comparison of direct hospital costs and length of stay for radical nephrectomy versus nephron-sparing surgery in the management of localized renal cell carcinoma. Urology 1999; 54: 994–8.

63. Poulakis V, Witzsch U, de Vries R et al. Quality of life after surgery for localized renal cell carcinoma: comparison between radical nephrectomy and nephron-sparing surgery. Urology 2003; 62: 814–20.

64. Marberger M, Pugh RC, Auvert J et al. Conservation surgery of renal carcinoma: the EIRSS experience. Br J Urol 1981; 53: 528–32.

65. Bazeed MA, Scharfe T, Becht E et al. Conservative surgery of renal cell carcinoma. Eur Urol 1986; 12: 238–43.

66. Carini M, Selli C, Barbanti G et al. Conservative surgical treatment of renal cell carcinoma: clinical experience and reappraisal of indications. J Urol 1988; 140: 725–31.

67. Morgan WR, Zincke H. Progression and survival after renal-conserving surgery for renal cell carcinoma: experience in 104 patients and extended followup. J Urol 1990; 144: 852–7; discussion 857–8.

68. Moll V, Becht E, Ziegler M. Kidney preserving surgery in renal cell tumors: indications, techniques and results in 152 patients. J Urol 1993; 150: 319–23.

69. Steinbach F, Stockle M, Muller SC. Conservative surgery of renal cell tumors in 140 patients: 21 years of experience. J Urol 1992; 148: 24–9; discussion 29–30.

70. Barbalias GA, Liatsikos EN, Tsintavis A et al. Adenocarcinoma of the kidney: nephron-sparing surgical approach vs. radical nephrectomy. J Surg Oncol 1999; 72: 156–61.

71. Zigeuner R, Quehenberger F, Pummer K et al. Long-term results of nephron-sparing surgery for renal cell carcinoma in 114 patients: risk factors for progressive disease. BJU Int 2003; 92: 567–71.

72. Van Poppel H, Bamelis B, Oyen R et al. Partial nephrectomy for renal cell carcinoma can achieve long-term tumor control. J Urol 1998; 160: 674–8.

73. McKiernan J, Yossepowitch O, Kattan MW et al. Partial nephrectomy for renal cortical tumors: pathologic findings and impact on outcome. Urology 2002; 60: 1003–9.

74. D'Armiento M, Damiano R, Feleppa B et al. Elective conservative surgery for renal carcinoma versus radical nephrectomy: a prospective study. Br J Urol 1997; 79: 15–19.

13

Future directions in nephron-sparing surgery

Alan M Nieder and Mark S Soloway

Over 40 years ago, Robson published his landmark study on renal cell carcinoma (RCC) which demonstrated improved survival when a more complete nephrectomy (i.e., radical) was performed.[1,2] While Robson's findings were dramatic, an even greater revolution in the management of RCC has subsequently occurred with the refinement and improvement in radiographic studies. During Robson's era most patients were diagnosed with RCC when they were symptomatic (e.g., palpable mass, abdominal pain, hematuria). Currently most renal masses are diagnosed incidentally, which has thus allowed a nephron-preserving approach to become routine practice.[3]

Multiple studies have demonstrated an equivalent disease-specific survival for patients who have undergone a total or partial nephrectomy.[4–7] More recently, laparoscopic partial nephrectomy has been developed as a less invasive technique for appropriate candidates.[8,9] Some have even used the DaVinci Robot to perform a laparoscopic partial nephrectomy.[10,11] The recent introduction of fibrin sealants has enhanced the surgeon's ability to rapidly achieve hemostasis and probably reduce urine extravasation.[12]

During the last decade even more minimally invasive approaches to small renal masses have been developed. Multiple centers have demonstrated the safety of cryo and radiofrequency ablation, either laparoscopic, open, or CT-guided, as a reasonable approach to the small renal mass.[13–15] Long-term survival data will be required to prove the utility of these even less invasive techniques for the treatment of RCC.

What is the future management of RCC? Clearly, major changes have occurred over the last two decades as improvements in surgical technique, imaging, and alternative ablative methods have been developed. Nevertheless, urologists still depend on radiographic criteria to diagnosis a renal mass and ultimately on postsurgical pathologic analyses to inform patients of

their prognosis. Nearly 60 years ago, Bell and Vermooten demonstrated that renal masses smaller than 3 cm have a minimal risk of metastasis and should be categorized as adenomas.[16,17] Yet, today, urologists operate on small renal masses and rarely recommend a biopsy.

Perhaps in the future, improved histochemical and pathologic analyses will provide urologists with better prognostic stratification of the small renal mass. Similarly, perhaps improved radiographic sensitivity will allow urologists to determine which patients can be followed. We already know that the annual size increase of a typical incidentally discovered small renal mass is minimal.[18–20] Small variations in size occur and small increases may not be significant.[21] In some centers up to 30% of renal masses are not malignant.[22,23] (In our center approximately 5% of tumors removed during partial nephrectomy are benign.)

Perhaps biopsy of the small renal mass will become common. Already, some centers have demonstrated the feasibility of diagnosing oncocytomas via percutaneous biopsy, thus obviating the need to remove the tumor.[24] Other centers are utilizing advanced gene expression analyses and fluorescence in-situ hybridization to differentiate an oncocytoma from RCC and subtype RCC.[25,26] Other novel immunohistochemical staining may provide further information regarding a tumor's biologic potential.[27] Furthermore, fine needle aspiration cytology may be able to identify renal lesions without the need for a larger needle biopsy.[28,29] Obviously, if lesions are known to be low-grade RCCs, adenomas, or oncocytomas, patients may be given a trial of observation prior to surgery.

Lastly, novel modalities may be utilized to treat RCC. High-intensity frequency ultrasound (HIFU) is a non-invasive treatment that has been demonstrated to successfully destroy renal tissue in experimental studies.[30] The benefit if successful, is that patients may be able to have their RCC ablated with no scars and minimal discomfort. While the published studies are preliminary, this modality may be successful in treating renal lesions.[31]

REFERENCES

1. Robson C. Radical nephrectomy for renal cell carcinoma. J Urol 1963; 89: 37–42.
2. Robson CJ, Churchill BM, Anderson W. The results of radical nephrectomy for renal cell carcinoma. J Urol 1969; 101: 297–301.
3. Jayson M, Sanders H. Increased incidence of serendipitously discovered renal cell carcinoma. Urology 1998; 51: 203–5.
4. Belldegrun A, Tsui KH, deKernion JB, Smith RB. Efficacy of nephron-sparing surgery for renal cell carcinoma: analysis based on the new 1997 tumor–node–metastasis staging system. J Clin Oncol 1999; 17: 2868–75.
5. Butler BP, Novick AC, Miller DP et al. Management of small unilateral renal cell carcinomas: radical versus nephron-sparing surgery. Urology 1995; 45: 34–40; discussion 40–1.
6. Lee CT, Katz J, Shi W et al. Surgical management of renal tumors 4 cm or less in a contemporary cohort. J Urol 2000; 163: 730–6.
7. Lerner SE, Hawkins CA, Blute ML et al. Disease outcome in patients with low stage renal cell carcinoma treated with nephron sparing or radical surgery. J Urol 1996; 155: 1868–73.
8. Lane BR, Gill IS. 5-Year outcomes of laparoscopic partial nephrectomy. J Urol 2007; 177: 70–4; discussion 74.
9. Permpongkosol S, Bagga HS, Romero FR et al. Laparoscopic versus open partial nephrectomy for the treatment of pathological T1N0M0 renal cell carcinoma: a 5-year survival rate. J Urol 2006; 176: 1984–8; discussion 1988–9.
10. Stifelman MD, Caruso RP, Nieder AM et al. Robot-assisted laparoscopic partial nephrectomy. JSLS 2005; 9: 83–6.
11. Kaul S, Laungani R, Sarle R et al. da Vinci-assisted robotic partial nephrectomy: technique and results at a mean of 15 months of follow-up. Eur Urol 2007; 51: 186–91; discussion 191–2.
12. Shekarriz B, Stoller ML. The use of fibrin sealant in urology. J Urol 2002; 167: 1218–25.
13. Gill IS, Remer EM, Hasan WA et al. Renal cryoablation: outcome at 3 years. J Urol 2005; 173: 1903–7.
14. Wyler SF, Sulser T, Ruszat R et al. Intermediate-term results of retroperitoneoscopy-assisted cryotherapy for small renal tumours using multiple ultrathin cryoprobes. Eur Urol 2007; 51(4): 971–9.
15. Park S, Anderson JK, Matsumoto ED et al. Radiofrequency ablation of renal tumors: intermediate-term results. J Endourol 2006; 20: 569–73.
16. Bell E A classification of renal tumors with observations of the frequency of the various types. J Urol 1938; 39: 238.
17. Vermooten V. Indications for conservative surgery in certain renal tumors. J Urol 1950; 64(2): 200–8.
18. Birnbaum BA, Bosniak MA, Megibow AJ et al. Observations on the growth of renal neoplasms. Radiology 1990; 176: 695–701.
19. Bosniak MA, Birnbaum BA, Krinsky GA et al. Small renal parenchymal neoplasms: further observations on growth. Radiology 1995; 197: 589–97.
20. Volpe A, Panzarella T, Rendon RA et al. The natural history of incidentally detected small renal masses. Cancer 2004; 100: 738–45.
21. Punnen S, Haider MA, Lockwood G et al. Variability in size measurement of renal masses smaller than 4 cm on computerized tomography. J Urol 2006; 176: 2386–90; discussion 2390.
22. Kutikov A, Fossett LK, Ramchandani P et al. Incidence of benign pathologic findings at partial nephrectomy for solitary renal mass presumed to be renal cell carcinoma on preoperative imaging. Urology 2006; 68: 737–40.
23. Snyder ME, Bach A, Kattan MW et al. Incidence of benign lesions for clinically localized renal masses smaller than 7 cm in radiological diameter: influence of sex. J Urol 2006; 176: 2391–5; discussion 2395–6.
24. Neuzillet Y, Lechevallier E, Andre M et al. Follow-up of renal oncocytoma diagnosed by percutaneous tumor biopsy. Urology 2005; 66: 1181–5.
25. Barocas DA, Mathew S, Delpizzo JJ et al. Renal cell carcinoma sub-typing by histopathology and fluorescence in situ hybridization on a needle-biopsy specimen. BJU Int 2006.
26. Rohan S, Tu JJ, Kao J et al. Gene expression profiling separates chromophobe renal cell carcinoma from oncocytoma and identifies vesicular transport and cell junction proteins as differentially expressed genes. Clin Cancer Res 2006; 12: 6937–45.
27. Rioux-Leclercq N, Delcros JG, Bansard JY et al. Immuno-histochemical analysis of tumor polyamines discriminates high-risk patients undergoing nephrectomy for renal cell carcinoma. Hum Pathol 2004; 35: 1279–84.
28. Crapanzano JP. Fine-needle aspiration of renal angiomyolipoma: cytological findings and diagnostic pitfalls in a series of five cases. Diagn Cytopathol 2005; 32: 53–7.
29. Sun W, McGregor DK, Ordonez NG et al. Fine needle aspiration cytology of a low grade myxoid renal epithelial neoplasm: a case report. Acta Cytol 2005; 49: 525–9.
30. Hacker A, Michel MS, Marlinghaus E et al. Extracorporeally induced ablation of renal tissue by high-intensity focused ultrasound. BJU Int 2006; 97: 779–85.
31. Illing RO, Kennedy JE, Wu F et al. The safety and feasibility of extracorporeal high-intensity focused ultrasound (HIFU) for the treatment of liver and kidney tumours in a Western population. Br J Cancer 2005; 93: 890–5.

Index

NB. Page numbers in *italic* denote figure and table legends